歯科衛生士

英語ワークブック

監修

山本 一世　　　　大阪歯科大学歯学部歯科保存学講座　教授

編著

藤田 淳一　　　　大阪歯科大学歯学部英語教室　教授

著

岡 隼人　　　　　大阪歯科大学歯学部英語教室　助教

寺島 雅子　　　　大阪歯科大学医療保健学部　助手／歯科衛生士

井村 和希　　　　井村歯科クリニック　院長

Julia Gadd　　　　英語講師

Brian Bachman　　大阪歯科大学歯学部英語教室　講師（非常勤）

表紙・イラスト

のんたろ

Special thanks to

Yuichi Hatada, Mutti, Chie Orita, Akiko Sowa, Kazuhiko Suese
Papageorgiou Dental Associates, The Smile Workx

協賛

株式会社モリタ、サンスター株式会社、ライオン株式会社（五十音順）

永末書店

序

　超高齢化社会を迎え、歯科医療を取り巻く状況も大きく変化しています。チーム医療・多職種連携が加速する中、歯科衛生士の役割は今後ますます大きくなってゆくことは間違いなく、医療従事者の一員としての役割を自覚し、より一層スキルを高めてゆくことが大切です。

　また 2019 年 12 月に確認された新型コロナウイルス感染症は瞬く間に世界中に拡散し、人々の日常を一変させましたが、足掛け 3 年にわたるコロナの蔓延もようやく終息の兆しが見えるようになり、外国人観光客の渡航制限も徐々に緩和されてきました。観光資源に富む日本ではインバウンドが回復するとともに、一度日本を離れていた外国人居住者たちも、再び来日することが予想されます。それに伴い外国人による医療機関の利用が増え、歯科医院に努める歯科衛生士が外国人の患者さんに対応しなければならない場面も出てくるでしょう。時には急患での突然の来院もあるかもしれません。そのような様々なケースに備えて、しっかりとした英語での対応ができることも、これからの時代に求められる歯科衛生士像のひとつではないでしょうか。

　この『歯科衛生士英語ワークブック』は、これまでも歯科医師や看護師向けの英会話ワークブックで実績のある大阪歯科大学のスタッフが、とくに歯科衛生士や歯科衛生士を目指して勉強している皆さんに、医療現場で役立てていただくことを目的とし、新時代のニーズを見据えて作られた実践的な歯科衛生士向けの英語教本です。テキストとともにスマートフォンで手軽に見ることができる動画が付いているので、無理なく楽しく、実践的な英会話を学ぶことができます。本書によって、皆さんが外国人の患者さんに英語で対応できる素敵な歯科衛生士となられることを期待し、ぜひ臨床の場で常備、必携されることをお勧めする次第です。

2022 年 12 月

大阪歯科大学　理事長・学長　川添堯彬

刊行によせて

　日本語が話せない外国の方が来院したら誰でも焦ります。しかし、外国人であっても歯科医療に関しては素人です。さらに痛みなどの症状や不安を抱えています。そのため複雑な構文や凝った表現、また難しい専門用語は不要です。つまり、基本的なフレーズさえ押さえておけば、語学が苦手な人でも十分に英語での対応ができます。

　本書では、100 本以上の動画を視聴し、ワークブック形式で歯科医院で外国人に対応するのに必要な英語のフレーズを身に着けることができます。外国人患者と意思疎通ができれば、歯科衛生士として一段ステップアップするとともに、今までに感じたことがない語学に対する自信が湧くでしょう。

2022 年 12 月

大阪歯科大学歯学部歯科保存学講座　教授　山本一世

大阪歯科大学歯学部英語教室　教授　藤田淳一

目次

本書の使い方

動画へのアクセス

スマートフォンに QR コードリーダーなどのアプリが事前にインストールされているか確認してください。スマートフォンでテキスト内に印刷されている QR コードを読み取ります。パスワード（**2023**）を入力していただきますと、そのレッスンの動画がまとめて表示されます。必要な動画を選んで再生してください。以下の URL（右記の QR コード）内にテキスト内のすべての動画があります。

http://vimeo.com/showcase/shikaeiseishiallvideos

まあこのワンポイントアドバイス

まあこ先生が歯科衛生士として日頃心掛けていることを英語でアドバイスしています。レッスン前に軽く読んで頭を「英語モード」に切り替えましょう。

1　Vocabulary

各レッスンのテーマに関連する用語です。これらの用語を英語及び日本語に訳して空欄に書き込みます。授業では、学生同士でペアを組みます。片方の学生は、テキストを見ながら各用語を読み上げます。もう一方の学生は、それに対して（テキストを見ず）素早く英語又は日本語に訳します。この練習方法をQuick Responseと呼び、英単語を目ではなく、耳で覚える練習です。

2　Brian's Pronunciation Practice　（動画付き）

Core Terms で取り上げられた単語をブライアン先生が発音します。動画を見ながら彼に続いて発音の練習をしましょう。

3　Brian's Pronunciation Tips　（動画付き）

日本人が特に苦手としている発音に焦点を当て、ブライアン先生が解説してくれています。動画を見て、下線部の発音に注意しながら、先生に続いてリピートしましょう。

4　Core Phrases

各レッスンのテーマに関連するフレーズです。Dialogs の歯科衛生士のセリフから抜粋したものです。きっちりと日本語に訳しましょう。ここでは歯科衛生士が使うであろう英語のフレーズを習得しましょう。

5　Quick Response　（動画付き）

上記4のフレーズでQuick Response の練習をします。動画を見ながら日本語に対する英訳を瞬時に言います。今までの英語の勉強は文字を見て覚えてきました。しかし、実際に外国人患者の対応をするときは、文字を当てにすることはできません。相手が発した英語を聞いて即座に反応しなければなりません。そこで通訳者の養成教育によく用いられるクィックレスポンスの練習をします。動画で読み上げられた日本語を聞いて即座に英語に訳す練習です。ポイントは、動画の音声に対して即座に反応することです。

6　Handy Phrases　（動画付き）

現場で言えたら便利なひとことです。動画を見て練習しましょう。

7　Workout with Julia　（動画付き）

ジュリア先生と、器具やオーラルケア用品の名称や現場で使う用語やフレーズなどの練習をしましょう。

8　Dialogs（動画付き）

現場での外国人患者の対応で起こりそうな場面を対話形式の動画にしています。まず動画を見て概要を理解してください。その後、再び動画を見ながらテキスト内の空欄を埋めます。空欄になっているのは外国人患者の返答として予測されるフレーズなので、しっかりと聞き取れるようにしましょう。

9　Patient Interview Drill　（動画付き）

巻末のPatient Interview Drill（p.75 ～）を切り取って使います。表面は歯科衛生士による患者への問診の動画を見て、問診表に患者による回答を日本語あるいは英語で書きとる課題です。裏面は表面の解答となっており、答え合わせ後に学生同士ペアになって、ロールプレイングの練習で使用することができます。クリップボードなどに挟んでご利用ください。

歯科衛生士
英語ワークブック

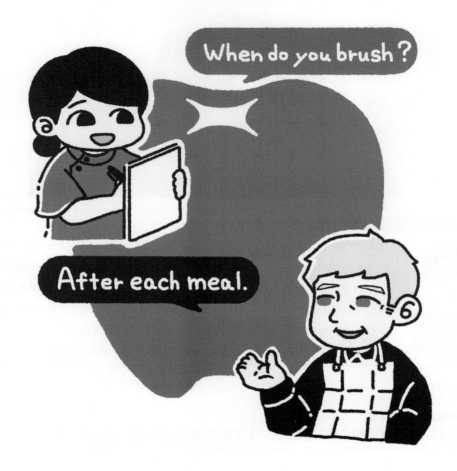

Lesson 1
Reception
受付

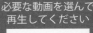

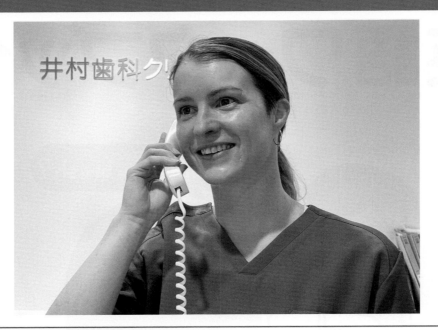

まあこのワンポイントアドバイス

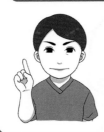

The receptionist is the first person that the patient comes into contact at the dental clinic. This encounter strongly influences the so-called first impression of the clinic. Keep in mind that the reason for the visit is usually pain, discomfort, or even anxiety toward their oral health. It is our job to help remove these problems and establish rapport. A smile and expression of empathy will help make that first impression a positive one.

1 Vocabulary
次の語を英語の場合は日本語に、日本語の場合は英語に直しなさい。

1．来院 　　　　　2．health insurance card 　　　　　3．fill out

4．form 　　　　　5．appointment 　　　　　6．gums

7．upper right 　　　　　8．swollen 　　　　　9．pain

10．right away 　　　　　11．分

2 Brian's Pronunciation Practice
動画の音声に続いて、リピートしなさい。

3 Brian's Pronunciation Tips
動画の音声に続いて、単語の発音練習をしなさい。

health	th の前後に u の音を入れて、ヘルスと発音しないように。
address	dd の後に o の音、ss の後に u の音を入れて、アドレスと発音しないように。
clinic	最初と最後の c の後に u の音を入れて、クリニックと発音しないように。

4 Core Phrases
次の英文を和訳しなさい。

1．May I have your name?

2．Do you have your health insurance card?

3．I will take a copy.

4．Please be seated.

5．Please fill out this form.

6．What seems to be the problem?

5 Quick Response
動画を見て、日本語に対する英語を瞬時に口頭で言いなさい。
瞬発力が大事です！

6 Handy Phrases
動画を見てとっさのひとことを確認しなさい。

「施術中に患者さんのスリッパがだんだん脱げそうになっていてお困りの時」のひとこと。

You may take your slippers off.（スリッパを脱いでもいいですよ。）

7 Workout with Julia
動画を見て、ジュリアの指示に従って英語で言いなさい。
その後、下の枠に答えを英語で書きなさい。

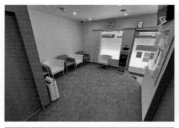

1

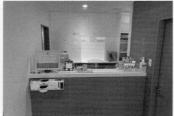

2

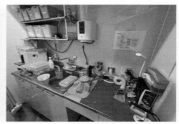

3

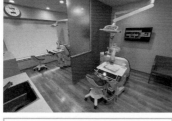

4

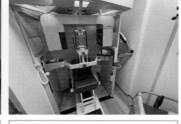

5

8 Dialogs
動画を見て各空欄に英単語１語を入れなさい。

Dialog 1：初めての来院

Patient:　　Hello. This is my (　　　　　　　　)(　　　　　　　　　　).

Hygienist: Hi! May I have your name?

Patient:　　Bachman. Brian Bachman.

Hygienist: Mr. Bachman, do you have a health insurance card?

Patient:　　(　　　　　　　)(　　　　　　　　)(　　　　　　　　).

Hygienist: Thank you. I will take a copy. Please be seated.

Patient:　　Thank you.

Hygienist: Mr. Bachman, here is your health insurance card.

Please fill out this form.

Patient:　Thank you.

Dialog 2：緊急の来院（アポなし）

Hygienist: Hello, Imura Dental Clinic.

Patient:　Hi. I don't have (　　　　　　)(　　　　　　).

Hygienist: Is this your first visit?

Patient:　Yes, it is.

Hygienist: May I have your name?

Patient:　My name is Brian Bachman.

Hygienist: What seems to be the problem, Mr. Bachman?

Patient:　My gums on the (　　　　　)(　　　　　) side are (　　　　　).

Hygienist: I see. Do you have any pain?

Patient:　Not much, but I have (　　　　　)(　　　　　).

Hygienist: Could you come right away?

Patient:　Yes. I'll be there in about (　　　　　)(　　　　　).

Hygienist: OK. We will be waiting for you.

9 Patient Interview Drill 1

▶巻末ドリルシート参照（p. 75-76）

a.　単語やフレーズの確認をしなさい。

| toothache | 歯痛 | something cold | 何か冷たいもの |
| painkillers | 痛み止め | rashes | 発疹 |

b.　動画を見て患者さんの回答を問診表に書き込みなさい。

c.　ペアを組んで歯科衛生士役と患者役に分かれて医療面接をしなさい。

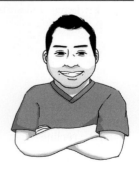

Lesson 2
Calling and Guiding
呼び出しと案内

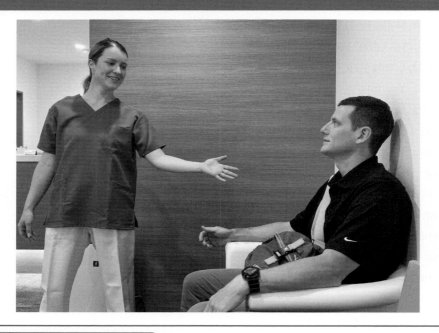

まあこのワンポイントアドバイス

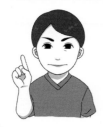

Imagine a first visit to a dental clinic. Do I change into slippers? Where do I hang my coat? What about my bag? Do I keep my slippers on when climbing onto the chair? These questions flash across the patient's mind. Worries about their cavity or swollen gums already lie heavily on their minds. There is no need to increase anxiety. Be sure to provide timely directions for a smooth guidance to the dental chair.

1 Vocabulary

次の語を英語の場合は日本語に、日本語の場合は英語に直しなさい。

1. leave
2. change to
3. スリッパ

4. bib
5. comfortable
6. need a hand

7. bend down
8. rack
9. watch your step

10. recline

2　Brian's Pronunciation Practice
動画の音声に続いて、リピートしなさい。

3　Brian's Pronunciation Tips
動画の音声に続いて、単語の発音練習をしなさい。

<u>s</u>lippers　最初の s の後に u の音を入れて、スリッパーズと発音しないように。
b<u>i</u>b　i を「イ」と「エ」の間で発音しましょう。
flo<u>ssi</u>ng　ssi を「シ」と発音しないように。「スィ」に近い発音です。

4　Core Phrases
次の英文を和訳しなさい。

1．Change to these slippers.

2．This way please.

3．I will put on your bib.

4．Are you comfortable?

5．Do you need a hand?

6．Watch your step.

5　Quick Response
動画を見て、日本語に対する英語を瞬時に口頭で言いなさい。
瞬発力が大事です！

6 Handy Phrases

動画を見てとっさのひとことを確認しなさい。

「患者さんが寒そうにしている時」のひとこと。

    Would you like a blanket?（ブランケットを掛けましょうか？）

〈応用編〉

    Let me fix your blanket?（ブランケットを上げますね。）

    Shall I remove the blanket?（ブランケットを取っておきましょうか？）

7 Workout with Julia

動画を見て、ジュリアの指示に従って英語で言いなさい。
その後、下の枠に答えを英語で書きなさい。

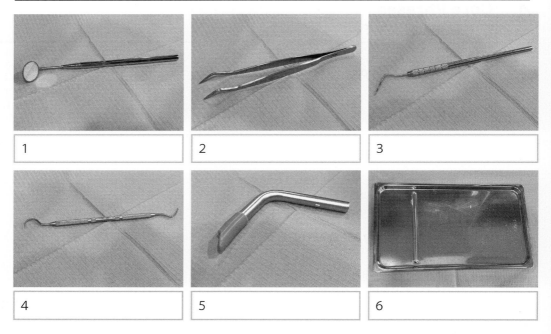

| 1 | 2 | 3 |
| 4 | 5 | 6 |

8 Dialogs

動画を見て各空欄に英単語1語を入れなさい。

Dialog 1：呼び出しと案内

Hygienist: You may leave your shoes here.

Patient: Sure.

Hygienist: Please change to these slippers.

Patient: Thank you.

Hygienist: Mr. Bachman?

Patient: Yes.

Hygienist: This way please.

Patient:　Where can I (　　　　　　　) my (　　　　　　　)?

Hygienist: You can put it here.

Hygienist: I will put on your bib.

　　　　　Are you comfortable?

Patient:　Yes, thank you.

Dialog 2：案内（患者さんが腰痛の場合）

Hygienist: Can you change to these slippers?

Patient:　I'll try.

Hygienist: What's wrong? Do you need a hand?

Patient:　I have a (　　　　　　　)(　　　　　　　).

　　　　　It hurts when I (　　　　　　　)(　　　　　　　).

Hygienist: Take your time. I'll put your shoes on the rack.

Patient:　Thanks.

Hygienist: This way please and watch your step.

　　　　　Please, sit here.

　　　　　Is it OK to recline?

Patient:　It's OK if you do it (　　　　　　　).

9　Patient Interview Drill 2

▶巻末ドリルシート参照 (p. 77-78)

a.　単語やフレーズの確認をしなさい。

a day　1 日に　　　　　　**spend ～ on …**　…に～を費やす

dental floss　フロス

b.　動画を見て患者さんの回答を問診表に書き込みなさい。

c.　ペアを組んで歯科衛生士役と患者役に分かれて医療面接をしなさい。

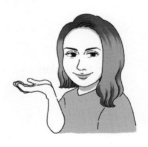

必要な動画を選んで
再生してください

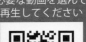

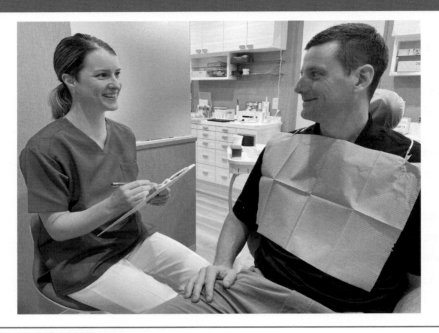

まあこのワンポイントアドバイス

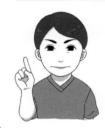

Patient interviews are important in obtaining information to determine the direction of the treatment. However, patients do not always tell the whole story. Some may be hesitant in sharing embarrassing information such as neglect of daily oral care due to laziness or economic reasons. Create an atmosphere that makes it easier for the patients to tell their story. Don't forget to brush up your communication skills.

1　Vocabulary
次の語を英語の場合は日本語に、日本語の場合は英語に直しなさい。

1．receive

2．治療

3．high blood pressure

4．薬

5．diabetes

6．blood sugar count

7．meal plan

8．exercise plan

9．feel sick

2　Brian's Pronunciation Practice
動画の音声に続いて、リピートしなさい。

3　Brian's Pronunciation Tips
動画の音声に続いて、単語の発音練習をしなさい。

pressure　pre が「プゥレ」とならないようにしましょう。

diabetes　betes の箇所を「ビィーティーズ」と伸ばすこと。形容詞は diabetic と発音が異なります。

receive　r と l の発音の違いに注意しましょう。

4　Core Phrases
次の英文を和訳しなさい。

1．Are you receiving any treatment now?

2．Are you taking any medication?

3．What is your blood pressure?

4．What is your blood sugar count?

5．Please let me know if you feel sick.

5　Quick Response
動画を見て、日本語に対する英語を瞬時に口頭で言いなさい。
瞬発力が大事です！

6 Handy Phrases
動画を見てとっさのひとことを確認しなさい。

「エプロンがズレた時」のひとこと。

Let me fix your bib.（エプロンのズレを直しますね。）

〈応用編〉

「エプロンが濡れた時」のひとこと。

Let me change your bib.（エプロンを交換します。）

7 Workout with Julia
歯科英語には一般用語（lay term）と専門用語（technical term）が
あります。今回は一般用語について勉強しましょう。

a. 動画を見て英語を書きとりなさい。

1		前歯
2		歯石
3		虫歯
4		乳歯
5		永久歯
6		歯茎
7		咬み合わせ
8		奥歯
9		矯正装置
10		親知らず

b. 動画を見て発音しなさい。

c. 動画を見て日本語から英語にクイックレスポンスしなさい。

8 Dialogs
動画を見て各空欄に英単語1語を入れなさい。

Dialog 1：医療面接（血圧）

Hygienist: Are you receiving any treatment now?

Patient:　　I go to the hospital for (　　　　　　　　)(　　　　　　　　　)(　　　　　　　　).

Hygienist: Are you taking any medication?

Patient:　　I take pills (　　　　　　　　)(　　　　　　　　) day.

Hygienist: What is your blood pressure on medication?

Patient:　　It is (　　　　　　　　) over (　　　　　　　　).

Hygienist: What is it without medication?

Patient:　　It is (　　　　　　　　) over (　　　　　　　　).

Dialog 2：医療面接（血糖値）

Hygienist: Are you receiving any treatment now?

Patient:　　I am receiving treatment for (　　　　　　　　).

Hygienist: What is your blood sugar count?

Patient:　　It was (　　　　　　　　) this morning.

Hygienist: Are you taking any medication?

Patient:　　No, I am on a meal plan and exercise plan.

Hygienist: Please let me know if you feel sick.

9　Patient Interview Drill 3　　　　　

▶巻末ドリルシート参照（p. 79-80）

a. 単語やフレーズの確認をしなさい。

　　slight pain　少しの痛み　　　　　　**severe pain**　激しい痛み

b. 動画を見て患者さんの回答を問診表に書き込みなさい。

c. ペアを組んで歯科衛生士役と患者役に分かれて医療面接をしなさい。

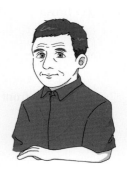

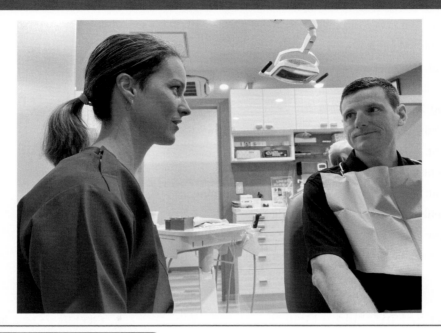

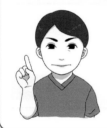
まあこのワンポイントアドバイス

Providing an effective oral care plan will definitely improve the oral health of your patients. However, the same instructions do not necessarily apply to each and every person. Patients have different backgrounds and daily habits that may influence their oral condition. Listen closely to what the patients say and apply what you have learned to form a set of instructions catered to each individual.

1 Vocabulary
次の語を英語の場合は日本語に、日本語の場合は英語に直しなさい。

1. brush	2. once or twice	3. mouthwash
4. コーヒー	5. throughout	6. swelling
7. bottom front	8. 痛む（h）	9. bleeding
10. tartar	11. otherwise	

2　Brian's Pronunciation Practice

動画の音声に続いて、リピートしなさい。

3　Brian's Pronunciation Tips

動画の音声に続いて、単語の発音練習をしなさい。

mouth　　マウス（mouse）と発音しないようにしましょう。

bottom　　ボトムではありません。o の音は a で発音しましょう。

tar<u>tar</u>　　ターターではありません。後ろの tar は ter と発音しましょう。

4　Core Phrases

次の英文を和訳しなさい。

1．How many times a day do you brush?

2．When do you brush your teeth?

3．Do you drink a lot of coffee, tea, or wine?

4．Where is the swelling?

5．When did the swelling start?

6．Do you have any pain?

7．Have you ever had your tartar removed?

8．Did you experience any problems then?

5　Quick Response

動画を見て、日本語に対する英語を瞬時に口頭で言いなさい。
瞬発力が大事です！

6 Handy Phrases
動画を見てとっさのひとことを確認しなさい。

スリーウェイシリンジを使うときのひとこと。

このように「I will」を言うことで患者さんに何をするのか事前に伝えることにができます。

I will spray some water. （水を吹きかけますね。）

I will blow some air. （空気を吹き付けますね。）

7 Workout with Julia

a. 動画を見て各名称を英語で書きとりなさい。

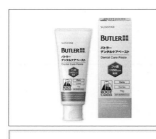

1

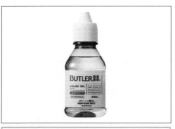

2

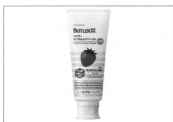

3

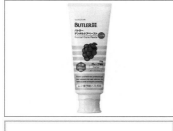

4

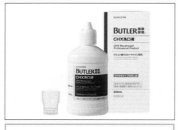

5

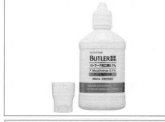

6

b. 動画を見て発音しなさい。

8 Dialogs
動画を見て各空欄に英単語1語を入れなさい。

Dialog 1：口腔ケアに関する医療面接

Hygienist: How many times a day do you brush?

Patient:　I would say (　　　　　　　　) or (　　　　　　　　).

Hygienist: When do you brush your teeth?

Patient:　In the (　　　　　　　　)...but when I am late for work, I just use (　　　　　　　　).

Hygienist: Do you brush at night?

Patient:　　Yes, I brush my teeth before (　　　　　　)(　　　　　　)

　　　　　　(　　　　　　　　) but I sometimes fall asleep after a night out drinking.

Hygienist: I see. Do you drink a lot of coffee, tea, or wine?

Patient:　　I drink a lot of (　　　　　　) throughout the day.

　　　　　　I sometimes have (　　　　　) with dinner.

Hygienist: Do you smoke?

Patient:　　No, I don't.

Dialog 2：症状に関する質問

Hygienist: Where is the swelling?

Patient:　　It is in the (　　　　　　)(　　　　　　).

Hygienist: When did the swelling start?

Patient:　　About (　　　　　)(　　　　　　) ago.

Hygienist: Do you have any pain?

Patient:　　It does not (　　　　　　). However, there is some (　　　　　)

　　　　　　when I (　　　　　　) my teeth.

Hygienist: Have you ever had your tartar removed at a dental clinic?

Patient:　　Yes, about 5 years ago.

Hygienist: Did you experience any problems then?

Patient:　　It was (　　　　　　) otherwise, no.

9 Patient Interview Drill 4

 ▶巻末ドリルシート参照（p. 81-82）

a. 単語やフレーズの確認をしなさい。

pay attention　注意を払う　　　　　　　**toothpick**　爪楊枝
pack　（タバコなどの）箱

b. 動画を見て患者さんの回答を問診表に書き込みなさい。

c. ペアを組んで歯科衛生士役と患者役に分かれて医療面接をしなさい。

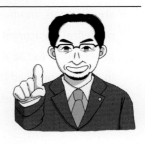

Dental Hygienists Around the World
1. Samoa / JICA Volunteers

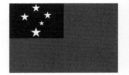

織田 千恵
JICA ボランティアとしてサモアで活動された織田千恵さんへの
インタビューをしました。

Q1. How did you become involved in JICA Volunteers?

After hearing about JICA Volunteers when I was working at the public health department, I wanted to do work in developing countries.

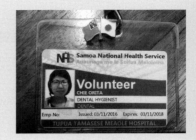

Q2. How was your English at that time? How did you prepare?

Honestly speaking, I was not very good at English. I started taking English conversation lessons and studied for the TOEIC test. After joining JICA Volunteers, there was an intensive English program. By 6 months after arriving at Samoa, I was able to communicate comfortably. I discovered it is important to speak out and not be ashamed of making mistakes.

Q3. Tell us a little about dentistry in Samoa.

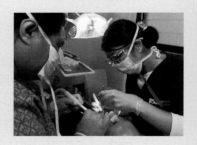

Dentists, dental therapists, dental technicians, and dental assistants make up the staff. Dental therapists conduct the same procedures as dental hygienists in Japan. In addition, they do all kinds of dental treatment except for root canal treatment and making dentures. The majority of cases in Samoa were restorative treatment for cavities. Tooth extraction was common. This is due to the lack of root canal treatment specialists. Dental therapists and hygienists conducted scaling procedures.

Q4. What kind of activities were you engaged in?

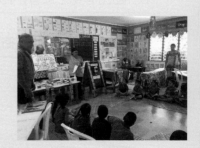

I did what I could do to improve the procedures for sterilization, management of dental tools, and assistance of dental treatment. I also offered advice concerning the procedures for scaling. There is a prevalence of diabetes in the region. I advised the staff to check the blood sugar count of the patients before taking on scaling procedures.

I also introduced brushing instructions for patients with periodontal disease. In addition, I organized a team to visit schools for dental checkups. In rural areas, there were many cases of oral care neglect.

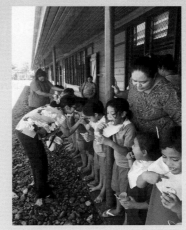

Q5. What did you learn from your experiences abroad?

When there is a lack of resources, it is important to discuss with the local staff and devise a plan together. Never force your ideas on anyone. Building a trusting relationship comes first. Then, you can offer your advice.

Q6. Can you share any interesting stories with us?

Wealthy people prefer gold coverings for their front teeth. In addition, many chew on smokeless tobacco in the region. That is why when they laugh, the inside of their mouths are all red.

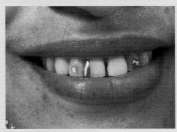

Q7. What is your present occupation?

I returned to my former job as faculty at a dental hygienist school. I often share my experiences abroad through my lectures. At graduate school, I obtained a master's degree based on my research on international oral health care activities.

Q8. Could you share some advice with the young dental hygienist students?

For safety reasons, always participate in overseas volunteer activities through JICA or NGOs. The experience abroad will open up new perspectives on the world. Do not hesitate if you do not have confidence in your English. Where there is a will, there is a way. I look forward to seeing more colleagues engaged in activities in developing countries.

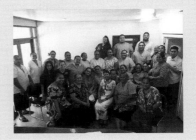

Vocabulary

developing countries	開発途上国	intensive English program	英語の集中プログラム
restorative treatment	保存修復治療	prevalence of diabetes	糖尿病患者が多い
oral care neglect	口腔ケアの放置	master's degree	修士号

Lesson 5
Basic Procedures
基本動作

必要な動画を選んで
再生してください

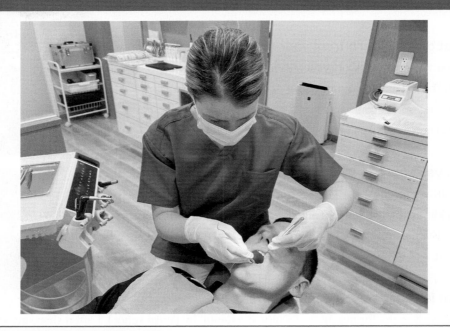

まあこのワンポイントアドバイス

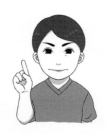

Imagine you are the patient sitting on the chair with your mouth open. When the dentist turns away to adjust his instruments, you would wonder if it is ok to close your mouth. This uncertainty may be uncomfortable to some patients. Do not leave the patients alone. Always be ready to provide timely instructions so the patients are exactly sure of what they need to do. Patients would be surprised if they are touched without any warning so be sure to tell them in advance.

1 Vocabulary
次の語を英語の場合は日本語に、日本語の場合は英語に直しなさい。

1. recline	2. 椅子	3. adjust
4. ヘッドレスト	5. 開けたままにする	6. bite down
7. rinse out	8. in a moment	9. 閉じる
10. 戻す	11. face down	12. comfortable

2　Brian's Pronunciation Practice
動画の音声に続いて、リピートしなさい。

3　Brian's Pronunciation Tips
動画の音声に続いて、単語の発音練習をしなさい。

open	オープンと発音しないように。
rinse	リンスと発音しないように。同じく return も注意しましょう。
comfortable	一気に発音しましょう。

4　Core Phrases
次の英文を和訳しなさい。

1．I will recline the chair.

2．I will adjust the headrest.

3．Open your mouth.

4．Open wide.

5．Keep your mouth open.

6．Bite down.

7．I will return the chair.

8．Rinse out your mouth.

9．The dentist will be with you in a moment.

10．Face down a little.

5　Quick Response
動画を見て、日本語に対する英語を瞬時に口頭で言いなさい。
瞬発力が大事です！

6 Handy Phrases
動画を見てとっさのひとことを確認しなさい。

「共感的態度」を示すときのひとこと。

Patient: I had a faver all last week. （先週はずっと熱が出ていました。）

Hygienist: Oh, that is too bad. / Oh, that is tough. （それはおつらいですね。）

So you held on all this time. （ああ、今まで我慢していたのですね。）

7 Workout with Julia

a. 動画を見てユニットの各部の名称を英語で書きとりなさい。

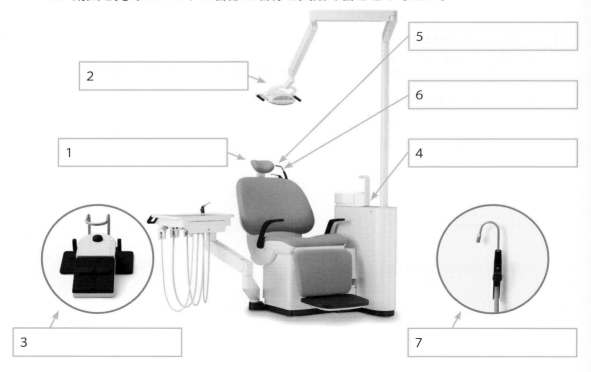

5

2

6

1

4

3

7

b. 動画を見ながら発音しなさい。

8 Dialogs
各指示文に対する患者の反応を注視しながら動画を見なさい。

Dialog 1：基本的な指示

Hygienist: I will recline the chair.

I will adjust the headrest.

Open your mouth, please.

Open wide.

Keep your mouth open, please.

Bite down, please.

I will return the chair.

Rinse out your mouth, please.

The dentist will be with you in a moment.

Patient:　Okay.

Dentist:　Hello!

Patient:　Hello.

Dialog 2：よくある場面

Hygienist: You may close your mouth.

...

Dentist:　Open your mouth, please.

...

Hygienist: I will return your chair.

Hygienist: Rinse out your mouth, please.

Patient:　Ooops.

...

Hygienist: I will change your bib.

Hygienist: Face down a little, please.

Hygienist: Are you comfortable?

Patient:　Yes, thank you.

9　Patient Interview Drill 5

▶巻末ドリルシート参照（p. 83-84）

a. 単語やフレーズの確認をしなさい。

chip　欠ける　　　　　　**granola**　グラノーラ（シリアル）

b. 動画を見て患者さんの回答を問診表に書き込みなさい。

c. ペアを組んで歯科衛生士役と患者役に分かれて医療面接をしなさい。

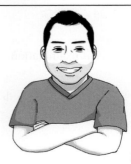

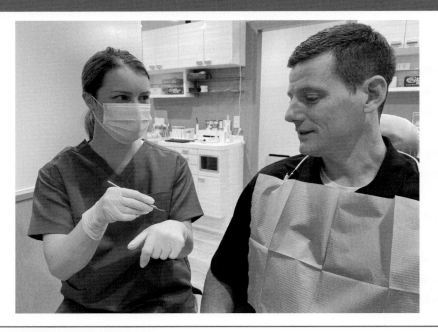

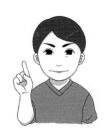

Since the probe looks like a needle, it may appear frightening to the patient. It would be a good idea to show the needle and playfully prick your gloved hand. The patient will notice that the tip is round and there is no need for alarm. Explain that if the gums are healthy, the probing would cause no pain. On the other hand, bleeding and pain are signs of inflammation. Tell the patients to let you know when they feel any pain. Appropriate information will ease any anxiety.

1 Vocabulary
次の語を英語の場合は日本語に、日本語の場合は英語に直しなさい。

1. pocket depth

2. condition

3. プローブ

4. 健康な

5. inflammation

6. 結果

7. examination

8. 表（c）

9. figures

10. ミリメートル

11. periodontal disease

24

2　Brian's Pronunciation Practice
動画の音声に続いて、リピートしなさい。

3　Brian's Pronunciation Tips
動画の音声に続いて、単語の発音練習をしなさい。

millim<u>e</u>ters	下線部のeは「イ」と発音します。メートルではありません。
de<u>pth</u>	pとthと子音が2つ重なっていますが、そこは一気に発音しましょう。
<u>po</u>cket	ポケットではありません。「ポ」よりは「パ」に近いです。

4　Core Phrases
次の英文を和訳しなさい。

1．I will check the pocket depth of your gums.

2．I will use this probe.

3．Please look at this chart.

4．These figures are the depth of your pockets.

5．Figures over 4mm have problems.

6．The red dots indicate bleeding.

5　Quick Response
動画を見て、日本語に対する英語を瞬時に口頭で言いなさい。
瞬発力が大事です！

6 Handy Phrases
動画を見てとっさのひとことを確認しなさい。

ヘッドレストに関してのひとこと。

I will adjust the headrest.（ヘッドレストを調整します。）

〈応用編〉

Would you like to take a rest?（ちょっと休憩されますか？）

I will return your headrest for a while.（少しの間、ヘッドレストを戻しますね。）

7 Workout with Julia
動画を見て、検査結果を患者さんに伝えましょう。

a．日本語を参考にそれぞれの空欄に英単語を入れなさい。

〈Case 1〉

1．あなたは深いポケットはありません。

You have (　　　　)(　　　　)(　　　　).

2．出血もありません。

There is (　　　　)(　　　　).

3．あなたの歯茎は健康です。

You have (　　　　)(　　　　).

歯周基本検査　2022.07.02　　name.

MOB		0	0	0	0	0	0	0	0	0	0	0	0	0	0	
PPD		3	3	3	3	3	2	2	2	2	3	3	3	3	3	
	8	7	6	5	4	3	2	1	1	2	3	4	5	6	7	8
PPD		3	3	3	2	2	2	2	2	2	3	3	3	3	3	
MOB		0	0	0	0	0	0	0	0	0	0	0	0	0	0	

〈Case 2〉

1．このポケットは 4mm です。

This pocket is (　　　)(　　　　)(　　　　).

2．出血があります。

There is (　　　　)(　　　　).

3．あなたは歯周炎になりかけています。

You are (　　　)(　　　　)(　　　　)(　　　　).

歯周基本検査　2022.07.02　　name.

MOB		0	0	0	0	0	0	0	0	0	0	0	0	0	0	
PPD		④	4	3	3	3	2	2	2	2	3	3	3	3	④	
	8	7	6	5	4	3	2	1	1	2	3	4	5	6	7	8
PPD		3	3	3	2	2	2	2	2	2	3	3	3	4	④	
MOB		0	0	0	0	0	0	0	0	0	0	0	0	0	0	

b．動画を見て答え合わせしなさい。

c．動画を見てジュリアに続いて英文を発音しなさい。

8 Dialogs
動画を見て各空欄に英単語1語を入れなさい。

Dialog 1：歯周検査の事前説明

Hygienist: We will check the pocket depth and condition of your gums.

Patient:　How will you do it?

Hygienist: I will use this probe.

Patient:　　Yikes! It (　　　　　　　)(　　　　　　　　)(　　　　　　　　) needle.
　　　　　　Will it hurt?
Hygienist: Take a look.
　　　　　　See, it isn't sharp at all.
Patient:　　Oh! That is a (　　　　　　　　).
Hygienist: If your gums are healthy, there will be no pain or bleeding.
Patient:　　(　　　　　　　)(　　　　　　　) there is pain or bleeding?
Hygienist: It is a sign of inflammation.
Patient:　　I see.

Dialog 2：歯周検査の結果説明

Hygienist: I will explain the results of the examination.
Patient:　　Okay.
Hygienist: Please take a look at this chart.
　　　　　　These figures are the depth of your pockets.
　　　　　　Those under 3mm are healthy. However, those over 4mm have problems.
Patient:　　(　　　　　　　)(　　　　　　　)(　　　　　　　　) problems are they?
Hygienist: There is the possibility of periodontitis or periodontal disease.
Patient:　　Oh, my gosh!
Hygienist: The deepest pocket is 6mm in the upper right.
　　　　　　There is also some swelling.
　　　　　　The red dots indicate bleeding from the examination.
Patient:　　I see.

9　Patient Interview Drill 6
▶巻末ドリルシート参照（p. 85-86）

a. 単語やフレーズの確認をしなさい。

normal	普通の	**order**	注文する
online	オンラインで	**cheap**	安い

b. 動画を見て患者さんの回答を問診表に書き込みなさい。

c. ペアを組んで歯科衛生士役と患者役に分かれて医療面接をしなさい。

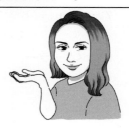

Lesson 7
Scaling
スケーリング

必要な動画を選んで
再生してください

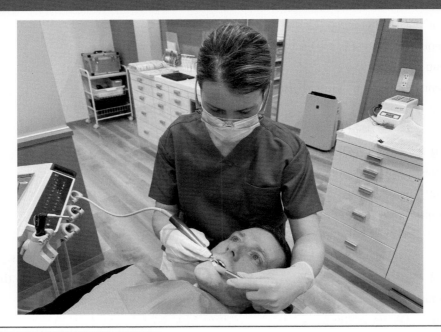

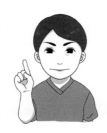

まあこのワンポイントアドバイス

Tartar gradually accumulates on the tooth surface so that people become used to its presence. After scaling, patients would look at the mirror and be surprised at the appearance of gaps between teeth. Also, the teeth themselves look longer than before and become sensitive. To prevent any unnecessary misunderstanding, explain the expected results in advance. Right after the treatment, tell the patient this is how their teeth are without tartar.

1 Vocabulary

次の語を英語の場合は日本語に、日本語の場合は英語に直しなさい。

1．plaque	2．sticky	3．film
4．bacteria	5．歯石（t）	6．ミネラル
7．saliva	8．combine	9．remaining
10．スケーラー	11．gaps	12．reminder

2　Brian's Pronunciation Practice
動画の音声に続いて、リピートしなさい。

3　Brian's Pronunciation Tips
動画の音声に続いて、単語の発音練習をしなさい。

scaling　　スケーリングとは発音しません。a は「エイ」と発音します。

sensitive　センシティブとは発音しません。下線部は「スィ」と発音します。

mirror　　ミラーとは発音しません。rr は巻き舌で発音します。

4　Core Phrases
次の英文を和訳しなさい。

1．It is a sticky film of bacteria.

2．Minerals in saliva combine with plaque.

3．I will remove it with this scaler.

4．Check with this mirror.

5．This is how your teeth should look.

6．We can send you a reminder by post.

5　Quick Response
動画を見て、日本語に対する英語を瞬時に口頭で言いなさい。
瞬発力が大事です！

6 Handy Phrases
動画を見てとっさのひとことを確認しなさい。

「患者さんの座る姿勢が崩れて、ズレ落ちそうになっている時」のひとこと。

Hygienist: **Please lift yourself up in the chair a little.**（少し姿勢を戻してくださいね。）

Patient:　Like this?（こんな感じ？）

Hygienist: Perfect.（完璧よ。）

7 Workout with Julia
今回は専門用語について勉強しましょう。

a.　動画を見て英語を書きとりなさい。

1		前歯
2		歯石
3		カリエス
4		乳歯
5		永久歯
6		歯肉
7		咬合
8		臼歯
9		矯正装置
10		智歯

b.　動画を見て発音しなさい。

c.　動画を見て日本語から英語にクイックレスポンスしなさい。

8 Dialogs
動画を見て各空欄に英単語１語を入れなさい。

Dialog 1：歯垢および歯石の説明

Patient:　What is (　　　　　　　　　)?

Hygienist: It is a sticky film of bacteria on your teeth.

Patient:　Can I remove it (　　　　　　　)?

Hygienist: Yes...with careful tooth brushing.

Patient:　Then, what is (　　　　　　)?

Hygienist: Minerals in your saliva combine with the remaining plaque and form tartar.

Patient:　Can I remove it myself?

Hygienist: No...I will remove it with this scaler.

Dialog 2：スケーリング後の会話

Hygienist: Check with this mirror.

Patient:　Oh my! What are all these (　　　　　　　)?

Hygienist: The gaps were filled with tartar.

Patient:　My teeth look (　　　　　　) than before.

Hygienist: That is because I removed all the tartar between your teeth and gums.

Patient:　I see.

Hygienist: This is how your teeth should look.

　　　　　When the gums become firm, the teeth may look longer.

Patient:　This means I should visit (　　　　　　)(　　　　　　　　).

Hygienist: Maybe so. We can send you a reminder by post every 6 months.

Patient:　That would be great!

9 Patient Interview Drill 7

▶巻末ドリルシート参照（p. 87-88）

a.　単語やフレーズの確認をしなさい。

crown　クラウン　　　　　　　　　　**fell out**　抜け落ちる

b.　動画を見て患者さんの回答を問診表に書き込みなさい。

c.　ペアを組んで歯科衛生士役と患者役に分かれて医療面接をしなさい。

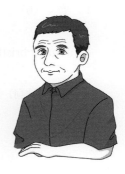

Lesson 8
Brushing Instructions
歯磨き指導

必要な動画を選んで再生してください

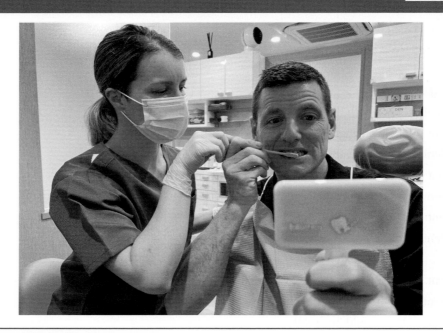

まあこのワンポイントアドバイス

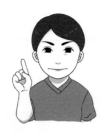

Some patients who neglect daily oral care brush their teeth right before visiting the clinic. This won't fool us! But don't blame the patient. Plaque disclosing is important in visualizing the areas missed during tooth brushing. Combine this with the information obtained from the patient interview. Tooth brushing instructions that better fit the patient's personality and lifestyle can be provided. Don't think of drastic changes. Go one step at a time.

1 Vocabulary
次の語を英語の場合は日本語に、日本語の場合は英語に直しなさい。

1．磨く（b）

2．強く

3．strokes

4．regular bristles

5．pen grip

6．softly

7．dye（動詞）

8．プラーク

9．stained red

10．gently

11．missed

2 Brian's Pronunciation Practice
動画の音声に続いて、リピートしなさい。

3 Brian's Pronunciation Tips
動画の音声に続いて、単語の発音練習をしなさい。

strokes　su・to・ro ではなく、str の発音を一気に発音しましょう。
brush　　ブラシとは発音しません。strokes 同様、母音を付けずに発音しましょう。
bristles　t は黙字です。

4 Core Phrases
次の英文を和訳しなさい。

1．Show me how you brush your teeth.

2．Choose a toothbrush with regular bristles.

3．Hold the toothbrush with a pen grip.

4．Brush softly with short strokes.

5．Your mouth will be stained red.

6．The red stains are the plaque you missed.

5 Quick Response
動画を見て、日本語に対する英語を瞬時に口頭で言いなさい。
瞬発力が大事です！

6 Handy Phrases
動画を見てとっさのひとことを確認しなさい。

チェアを離れるときのひとこと。
I'll be back. （すぐに戻ります。）

7 Workout with Julia
動画を見て、次の指示に従って歯磨き指導の練習をしなさい。

a. ジュリアの指示に従ってまあこ先生がブラッシングをしますので、確認しなさい。

b. ジュリアに続いて以下の文を発音練習しなさい。

1. Choose a toothbrush with regular bristles.
2. Hold the toothbrush with a pen grip.
3. Apply at a 90 degree angle.
4. Brush with short strokes.
5. Brush the outer surface of the teeth.
6. Brush the inner surface of the teeth.
7. Brush the chewing surface of the teeth.

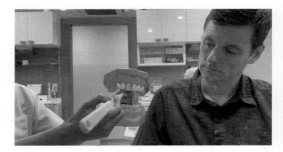

c. 上の英文に合わせて動作の練習をしなさい。

8 Dialogs
動画を見て内容を確認しなさい。

Dialog 1：歯磨き指導

Hygienist: Would you show me how you always brush your teeth?

Patient:　Sure.

Hygienist: Okay. You can stop.
　　　　　 You seem to brush too strongly.

Patient:　Really?!

Hygienist: Also, your strokes are too large.
　　　　　 Here, I will explain how to brush your teeth.
　　　　　 Choose a toothbrush with regular bristles like this.
　　　　　 Hold the toothbrush with a pen grip...like you did before.

Patient:　This way?

Hygienist: Very good.

Here, let me try it on you.

Brush softly with short strokes in this way.

Dialog 2：染め出し

Hygienist: I will dye the plaque you missed when brushing.

Patient:　OK.

Hygienist: Your mouth will be stained red.

Patient:　Stained?

Hygienist: Are you meeting anyone after this?

Patient:　Fortunately, no.

...

Hygienist: Rinse out your mouth gently.

Please check with this mirror.

The red stains are the plaque you missed when brushing.

Patient:　Oh my gosh!

9 Patient Interview Drill 8

▶巻末ドリルシート参照（p. 89-90）

a. 単語やフレーズの確認をしなさい。

vary　変わる　　　　manual　手動の（普通の）

powered　電動の　　　office　職場

b. 動画を見て患者さんの回答を問診表に書き込みなさい。

c. ペアを組んで歯科衛生士役と患者役に分かれて医療面接をしなさい。

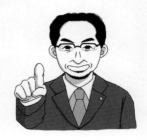

Dental Hygienists Around the World

2. Boston

Papageorgiou Dental Associates
(959 WORCESTER ST, NATICK, MA 01760)

ボストン郊外の Papageorgiou 歯科医院にお勤めの歯科衛生士さんに
アンケートに回答していただきました。

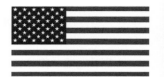

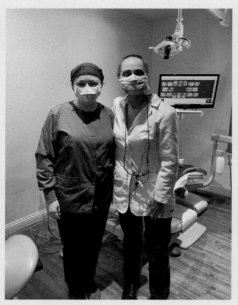

Hygienist and dentist

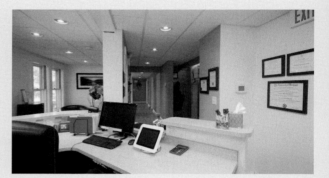

Reception

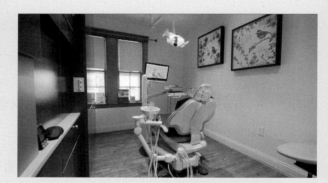

Treatment room

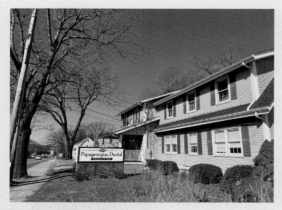

View from the front

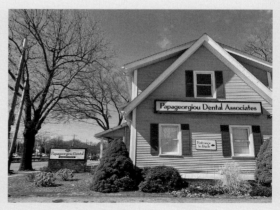

View from the parking lot

1. What kind of staff are working at private dental clinics in the US?

Doctor, Assistant, Front desk, Hygienist - (sometimes a separate manager)

2. What would be an average day at work? (daily schedule for hygienists)

Hygiene appointments between 45 and 60 minutes -

3. Do patients make appointments directly with you? or does the clinic arrange this?

Sometimes, but mostly with the front desk in case they need to make a payment

4. What kind of procedures/treatment do hygienists in the US conduct? For example, are they allowed to give local anesthetic injections?

regular dental cleanings, scaling and root planing, fluoride - Yes for local as long as they are certified

5. Can hygienists open their own clinics? If so, what kind of operations would they be? (such as location, hired staff, pricing)

Not in Massachusetts -

6. How do you balance your work and private time?

most hygienists work part time

7. What is the wage for hygienists in the US?

$40-50/ hour in Massachusetts - vary by location

8. What kind of fringe benefits are available?

Health insurance and 401K for full time employees

9. How many holidays do you get?

Five - for full time employees

10. How many years of schooling is necessary?

Two

11. Do you have a national board examination for hygienists?

Yes

Vocabulary

401K　資金を積み立て運用して資産を築く年金制度

Lesson 9
Stain Removal
ステイン除去

必要な動画を選んで再生してください

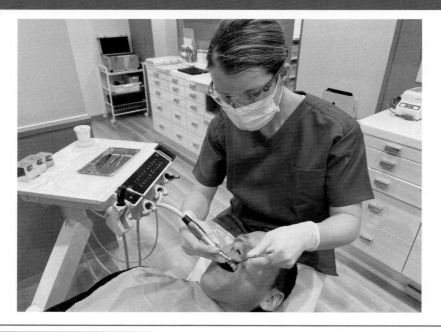

まあこのワンポイントアドバイス

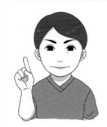

At the start, have the patient check their stains in the mirror. Tell them to run their tongue along the rough surfaces. After the stain removal, repeat the same procedure. The patient will sense the difference. Eating habits and drinking habits have a strong effect on tooth stains. This is why some patients require stain removal at shorter intervals. Encourage the patient to visit the clinic for regular cleaning.

1 Vocabulary
次の語を英語の場合は日本語に、日本語の場合は英語に直しなさい。

1．経験する

2．stain removal

3．remove

4．raise

5．smooth

6．鏡

7．違い

8．cut down on

9．every ～ months

10．tips

2 Brian's Pronunciation Practice
動画の音声に続いて、リピートしなさい。

3 Brian's Pronunciation Tips
動画の音声に続いて、単語の発音練習をしなさい。

trouble　子音が重なる tr の発音に注意しましょう。t の後に o を入れてトラブルと発音しないように。

coffee　コーヒーとは発音しません。ff は「ヒー」ではなく、「フィー」と発音します。

months　子音が重なる ths の発音に注意しましょう。

4 Core Phrases
次の英文を和訳しなさい。

1．Have you experienced stain removal before?

2．Did you experience any trouble?

3．I will remove your stains.

4．Please raise your left hand if it hurts.

5．Visit us every 6 months.

6．I will give you some brushing tips.

5 Quick Response
動画を見て、日本語に対する英語を瞬時に口頭で言いなさい。
瞬発力が大事です！

6 Handy Phrases

動画を見てとっさのひとことを確認しなさい。

「安心させる」ひとこと

Your treatment is over.（治療が終わりましたよ。）

7 Workout with Julia

a. 動画を見て各名称を英語で書きとりなさい。

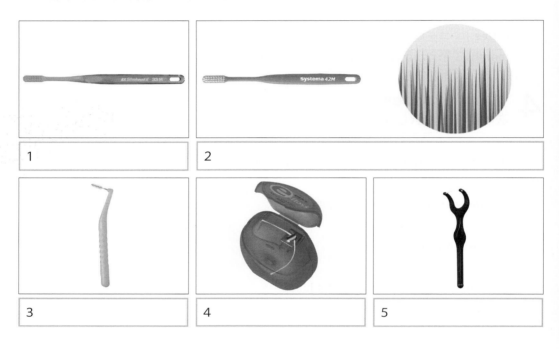

b. もう一度動画を見て発音しなさい。

8 Dialogs

動画を見て各空欄に英単語1語を入れなさい。

Dialog 1：ステイン除去前の会話

Hygienist: Have you experienced stain removal before?

Patient:　（　　　　　　　）, （　　　　　　　）（　　　　　　　）.

Hygienist: Did you experience any trouble?

Patient:　（　　　　　　　）, （　　　　　　　）（　　　　　　　）.

Hygienist: Now, I will remove your stains.

Please raise your left hand if it hurts.

Open your mouth.

Dialog 2：ステイン除去後の会話

Hygienist: We are finished.

Please rinse out your mouth.

Patient:　My teeth (　　　　　　　) so (　　　　　　　).

Hygienist: Please check with this mirror.

Patient:　Wow! What a difference.

Maybe I should (　　　　　)(　　　　　　)(　　　　　) coffee.

Hygienist: That wouldn't be necessary.

Visit us once every 6 months.

I will give you some brushing tips too.

Patient:　Great!

9　Patient Interview Drill 9

▶巻末ドリルシート参照（p. 91-92）

a.　単語やフレーズの確認をしなさい。

no matter how　どれだけ〜しても　　　　**right after**　すぐ後に

weekends　週末

b.　動画を見て患者さんの回答を問診表に書き込みなさい。

c.　ペアを組んで歯科衛生士役と患者役に分かれて医療面接をしなさい。

d.　同じペアで裏面を使ってロールプレイングをしてみましょう。
　　終わったら交代しましょう。

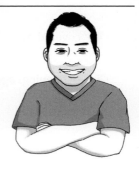

Lesson 10
Teeth Whitening
ホワイトニング

必要な動画を選んで
再生してください

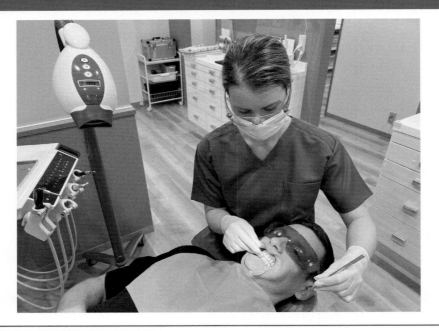

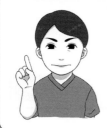

まあこのワンポイントアドバイス

Good counseling directly links to patient satisfaction. Here are some of the points to be explained. First, since whitening is not covered by health insurance, the patient will have to pay more than some other types of treatment. Second, the procedures can be conducted at the dental clinic, at home, or a combination of both locations. Third, during the treatment, there are restrictions in diet. Fourth, be sure to obtain consent.

1 Vocabulary
次の語を英語の場合は日本語に、日本語の場合は英語に直しなさい。

1. 白くなる

2. take a look

3. whitening treatment

4. covered by

5. consent form

6. mouth opening device

7. (whitening) agent

8. 光を当てる

9. remove

2 Brian's Pronunciation Practice
動画の音声に続いて、リピートしなさい。

3 Brian's Pronunciation Tips
動画の音声に続いて、単語の発音練習をしなさい。

agent　　　エーと伸ばさずに、エイジェントと発音しましょう。

whitening　ホではなく。ワと発音しましょう。

insurance　インシュランスとは発音しません。アクセントの位置に注意しましょう。

4 Core Phrases
次の英文を和訳しなさい。

1．There are individual differences.

2．You need to sign a consent form.

3．I will put in a mouth-opening device.

4．I will apply the whitening agent to your teeth.

5．I will shine light on your teeth.

6．You may close your eyes.

7．I will remove the agent.

5 Quick Response
動画を見て、日本語に対する英語を瞬時に口頭で言いなさい。
瞬発力が大事です！

6 Handy Phrases
動画を見てとっさのひとことを確認しなさい。

ひざ掛けがずれたときのひとこと。

Let me fix your blanket. （ひざ掛けを直しましょう。）

7 Workout with Julia

a． 英文を参考に空欄を埋めなさい。

1． Please avoid food and drinks that cause stains such as curry, chocolate, and coffee.
色のつく物は（　　　　　　　　　　）。例えば、カレー、チョコレート、コーヒー。

2． Please avoid high-acid food such as citrus, dressing, and cola.
酸性の食べ物は（　　　　　　　　）。
例えば、（　　　　　　　　　）、ドレッシング、コーラ。

3． There may be a recurrence of pain. Call us if it gets worse.
痛みが（　　　　　　　　）することもあります。
（　　　　　　　　）連絡ください。

4． Relapse of color will occur.
色の（　　　　　　　　　　）は起こります。

b． 動画を見て次の英文を発音しなさい。

1． Please avoid food and drinks.
2． Please avoid high-acid food.
3． There may be a recurrence of pain.
4． Relapse of color will occur.

8 Dialogs
Dialog 1は動画を見て各空欄に英単語1語を入れなさい。
Dialog 2は動画を見て内容を確認しなさい。

Dialog 1：ホワイトニングの相談
Patient:　No matter how much I brush, my teeth do not (　　　　　　　)(　　　　　　　).
Hygienist: Let's take a look.

Hygienist: They are not surface stains.

Patient:　What should I do?

Hygienist: You may need whitening treatment.

Patient:　I see. (　　　　　　　　)(　　　　　　　　) will my teeth become?

Hygienist: There are individual differences.

In most cases, they will become whiter.

Patient:　OK. Let's (　　　　　　　)(　　　　　　　).

Hygienist: May I remind you that it is not covered by insurance.

Also you need to sign a consent form.

Patient:　No problem!

Dialog 2：ホワイトニング治療

Hygienist: Please put on this eye guard.

I will put in a mouth-opening device.

I will apply the whitening agent to your teeth.

Do not bite down, please.

I will shine light on your teeth.

You may close your eyes.

Now, I will remove the agent.

Rinse out your mouth, please.

Please check with this mirror.

Patient:　Oh, amazing!

9　Patient Interview Drill 10

▶巻末ドリルシート参照（p. 93-94)

a.　単語やフレーズの確認をしなさい。

filling　詰め物　　　　　　　　**swallow**　呑み込む

a while ago　少し前に

b.　動画を見て患者さんの回答を問診表に書き込みなさい。

c.　ペアを組んで歯科衛生士役と患者役に分かれて医療面接をしなさい。

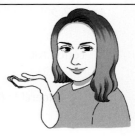

Lesson 11

Fluoride Application
フッ化物塗布

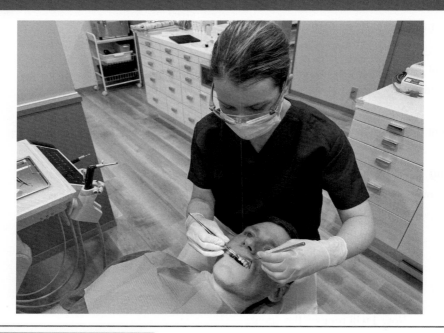

まあこのワンポイントアドバイス

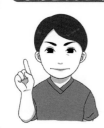

Fluoride strengthens the teeth and helps prevent cavities. Solutions, foam, gels, toothpaste, floss, and mouthwash containing fluoride are available. However, applying fluoride does not mean that you will not get any cavities. In addition, high doses may lead to fluoride toxicity. It is necessary to explain the proper usage to the patients.

1 Vocabulary

次の語を英語の場合は日本語に、日本語の場合は英語に直しなさい。

1. advantages

2. フッ化物

3. application

4. リスク

5. disadvantages

6. allergic reaction

7. cotton rolls

8. blow air on 〜

9. refrain from 〜

10. be vulnerable to 〜

11. 定期検診

2　Brian's Pronunciation Practice
動画の音声に続いて、リピートしなさい。

3　Brian's Pronunciation Tips
動画の音声に続いて、単語の発音練習をしなさい。

fluoride　　フルオーライドとは発音しません。u はほぼ発音しません。

vulnerable　v の音は日本人は苦手とされています。バではなく、ヴァと発音しましょう。

apply　　　アプリーではなく、アプライと発音しましょう。

4　Core Phrases
次の英文を和訳しなさい。

1．Fluoride makes your teeth stronger.

2．It doesn't mean you won't get cavities.

3．I will put some cotton rolls behind your lips.

4．I will blow air on your teeth.

5．I will apply fluoride to your teeth.

6．Please sit still for a few minutes.

5　Quick Response
動画を見て、日本語に対する英語を瞬時に口頭で言いなさい。
瞬発力が大事です！

6 Handy Phrases
動画を見てとっさのひとことを確認しなさい。

歯科医が途中でチェアを離れたときのひとこと。

Wait a moment please.（少しお待ちください。）

7 Workout with Julia
フッ化物塗布を自宅でする際の注意事項。動画を見て空欄を埋めなさい。

1． Use (　　　　　　) (　　　　　　　　) (　　　　　　　　　).
2． The dosage is (　　　　　　　)mL for preschoolers.
3． The dosage is (　　　　　　　)mL for elementary school children or older.
4． Rinse thoroughly for (　　　　　　　) seconds and spit out.
5． Rinse (　　　　　　) (　　　　　　　) to avoid swallowing.
6． Best used (　　　　　　　) (　　　　　　).
7． Use under (　　　　　　　) (　　　　　　).
8． Best used within (　　　　　　) (　　　　　　).
9． Swallowing (　　　　　　) (　　　　　　) (　　　　　　　)immediate poisoning.
10． (　　　　　　) (　　　　　　　　) drinking or eating for 30 minutes.

8 Dialogs
動画を見て各空欄に英単語1語を入れなさい。

Dialog 1：フッ化物塗布前の会話

Patient:　What are the (　　　　　　　　) of fluoride application?

Hygienist: Fluoride makes your teeth stronger.

Patient:　So it reduces the (　　　　　　　) of (　　　　　　　)?

Hygienist: Yes. However, it doesn't mean you won't get cavities.

Patient:　Okay.

Hygienist: Tooth brushing is important.

Patient:　Are there any (　　　　　　　)?

Hygienist: Sometimes, there are allergic reactions. However, it is rare.

Patient:　I see.

Dialog 2：フッ化物塗布の施術と術後の指導

Hygienist: Open your mouth, please.

　　　　　I will put some cotton rolls behind your lips.

　　　　　I will blow air on your teeth.

　　　　　Now I will apply fluoride to your teeth.

　　　　　Please sit still for a few minutes.

　　　　　We are finished.

Patient:　　When can I (　　　　　　　　)(　　　　　　　　)?

Hygienist: Please refrain from eating or drinking for 30 minutes.

Patient:　　(　　　　　　　　)(　　　　　　　　) should I get fluoride application?

Hygienist: Your teeth are vulnerable to cavities...maybe once every 6 months.

Patient:　　So at the same time as my (　　　　　　　)(　　　　　　　)?

Hygienist: Yes, certainly.

9　Patient Interview Drill 11

▶巻末ドリルシート参照（p. 95-96）

a.　単語やフレーズの確認をしなさい。

---

recommended　推奨される　　　　　　　　grip　持ち手

stuck　詰まる

b.　動画を見て患者さんの回答を問診表に書き込みなさい。

---

c.　ペアを組んで歯科衛生士役と患者役に分かれて医療面接をしなさい。

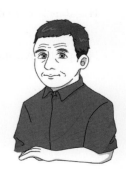

X-ray
エックス線写真（撮影）

必要な動画を選んで
再生してください

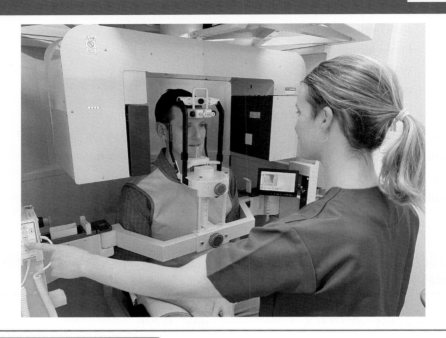

まあこのワンポイントアドバイス

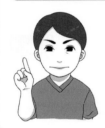

Dental hygienists do not operate the controls to take x-rays. However, it is our job to guide and set up the patient before the dentist presses the button. This will ensure a smooth and safe procedure. Some patients have feelings of anxiety towards x-rays. This may especially be the case for pregnant women. Acquire proper knowledge about x-rays so that you can guide the patients smoothly.

1　Vocabulary

次の語を英語の場合は日本語に、日本語の場合は英語に直しなさい。

1．エックス線写真（撮影）	2．worried	3．exposure
4．protective apron	5．重い	6．lead lining
7．chin	8．bite on	9．adjust
10．高さ	11．remain still	12．rotating

2 Brian's Pronunciation Practice
動画の音声に続いて、リピートしなさい。

3 Brian's Pronunciation Tips
動画の音声に続いて、単語の発音練習をしなさい。

apron　　a は「エ」ではなく、「エイ」と発音しましょう。

lead　　同じ綴りでも、導くの「リード」ではなく、鉛は「レッド」です。

still　　i は「イ」と「エ」の間の発音で伸ばさず短く発音しましょう。

4 Core Phrases
次の英文を和訳しなさい。

1．We need to take an x-ray.

2．X-ray exposure is very small.

3．Put on this protective apron.

4．Place your chin on this.

5．I will adjust the height.

6．Please remain still when the machine is rotating.

5 Quick Response
動画を見て、日本語に対する英語を瞬時に口頭で言いなさい。
瞬発力が大事です！

6 Handy Phrases

動画を見てとっさのひとことを確認しなさい。

治療が終わったと伝えるときのひとこと。

We are finished. I will take off your bib. （もう終わりましたよ。エプロン外しますね。）

7 Workout with Julia

動画を見て、それぞれの機器の使用目的を聞き取り、空欄を埋めなさい。

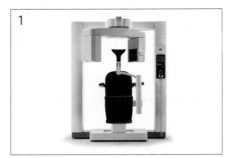

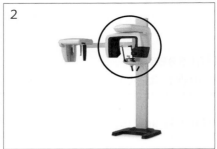

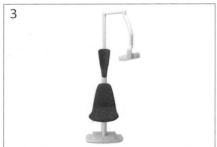

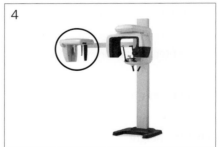

1．This is the cone beam CT.

It takes (　　　　　　　　　　)(　　　　　　　　　　　　　).

2．This is the panorama CT.

It takes 2D images of (　　　　　　　　)(　　　　　　　　　　).

3．This is the intraoral radiograph.

It takes 2D images of (　　　　　　　　)(　　　　　　　　　　).

4．This is cephalo radiograph.

It takes 2D images for (　　　　　　　　)(　　　　　　　　　　).

8 Dialogs

動画を見て各空欄に英単語1語を入れなさい。

Dialog 1：患者を安心させる

Hygienist: We need to take an x-ray to check your cavity.

Patient:　Is it (　　　　　　　　)(　　　　　　　　)?

Hygienist: Yes, why?

Patient:　I am a bit (　　　　　　　　) about (　　　　　　　　).

Hygienist: I see. Actually, x-ray exposure is very small.

Patient:　Oh, really!

Dialog 2：エックス線撮影での指示

Hygienist: Please put on this protective apron.

Patient:　It is a bit (　　　　　　　　).

Hygienist: Yes, it has lead lining.

　　　　　Please sit here.

Patient:　OK.

Hygienist: Place your chin on this and bite on this.

Patient:　(　　　　　　　　)(　　　　　　　　)?

Hygienist: Yeah.

Hygienist: I will adjust the height and the position of your head.

　　　　　Please remain still when the machine is rotating.

9 Patient Interview Drill 12

▶ 巻末ドリルシート参照（p. 97-98）

a. 単語やフレーズの確認をしなさい。

swollen　腫れた　　　　　　　　Oops　しまった

b. 動画を見て患者さんの回答を問診表に書き込みなさい。

c. ペアを組んで歯科衛生士役と患者役に分かれて医療面接をしなさい。

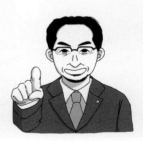

Dental Hygienists Around the World
3. Brisbane

The Smile Workx
(48 Mary St. Noosaville, QLD 4566, Australia)
Julia さんが地元のブリスベインにてかかりつけの歯科医院でインタビューをしました。

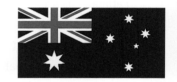

Q1. What kind of staff work at private dental clinics in Australia?

In normal private dental practice settings, we have of course, the dentist, chairside dental assistant, and another assistant that might help in sterilization of the instruments, reception, and a practice manager as well. Some dentists prefer to have dental hygienists or oral health therapists to help increase efficiency.

Q2. What would be an average day at work for a hygienist?

A hygienist would work Monday through Friday, 38 hours per week so 7 to 8 hours every day.

Q3. What is the hygienist's daily schedule?

Most of the hygienists work by themselves which means they may not have a dental assistant helping them because their main task is to perform oral hygiene on the patients which is cleaning their teeth and polishing their teeth. They may also do teeth whitening, take impressions, and take photos.

Q4. How do patients make appointments?

99% of the patients make appointments by phone. When someone is in pain, they might walk in. Otherwise, most of the patients have appointments booked well in advance. Some patients make their 6 month regular checkup and clean visits well in advance. They would have their cleaning done and at the front desk, they would make their next appointment.

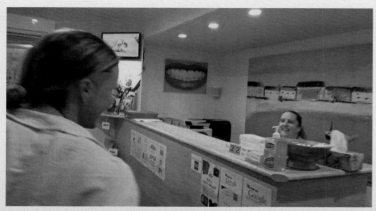

Receptionist

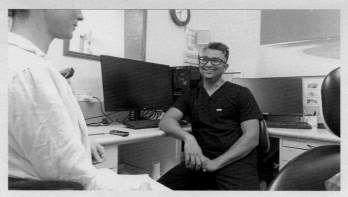

Dr. Chintan Soni

Q5. What kind of procedures or treatments do hygienists in Australia conduct?

Hygienists have to work under the dentist registration. They cannot perform any of the procedures in the absence of the dentist. So, the dentist has to be there all the time as a supervisor. Under the supervision of the dentist, they can do teeth cleaning, also it could be a deep clean of the gums in the case of gum disease, local anesthesia, teeth whitening, taking impressions, taking x-rays, making some appliance like night guard trays and that sort of thing.

Q6. Can hygienists open their own clinics?

No. They cannot work independently. They need to have supervision of a dentist.

Q7. What is the wage for hygienists in Australia?

The starting wage would be about 30 dollars per hour. As they get more experience, their wages may go up. In some practices, they may be offered a commission as well. So if they are performing very well, they might get some bonus commission on top of their basic wage.

Q8. How many holidays do you get?

On the average, we try to have a 3 to 4 week holiday a year.

Q9. How many years of schooling is necessary for dentists and hygienists?

For hygienists, it is 3 years. For the dentist, it is 5 years.

Vocabulary

increase efficiency　効率を上げる	walk in　急患で来院する
well in advance　十分前もって	in the absence of ～　～の不在
under the supervision of ～　～の監修のもと	starting wage　初任給
commission　手当	

Lesson 13
Impression Taking
印象採得

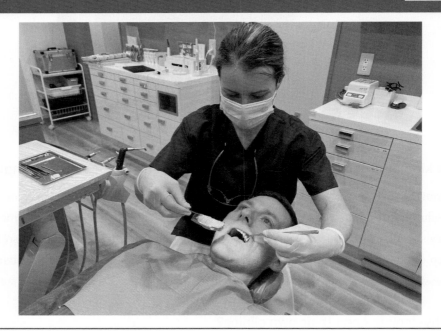

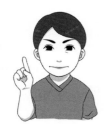

まあこのワンポイントアドバイス

Impression taking can be a nightmare for some patients. The smell of the alginate impression material, the sensation of your mouth filling up, and the strong reaction caused by gag reflex can make impression taking an excruciating experience. Just thinking about all this can lead to anxiety building up in the patients. It is necessary for us to make the patients feel relaxed and do the procedure as smoothly and quickly as possible.

1 Vocabulary

次の語を英語の場合は日本語に、日本語の場合は英語に直しなさい。

1．impression	2．model	3．冷たく感じる
4．息をする	5．through your nose	6．harden
7．トレー	8．retch	9．hum
10．drool		

2 Brian's Pronunciation Practice
動画の音声に続いて、リピートしなさい。

3 Brian's Pronunciation Tips
動画の音声に続いて、単語の発音練習をしなさい。

model　oは「オ」ではなく、「ア」に近い発音をしましょう。

tray　トレーとは発音せず、下線部分を一気に発音しましょう。

hum　uは口の上で発音するのではなく、口の下で発音するイメージです。

4 Core Phrases
次の英文を和訳しなさい。

1．I will take an impression.

2．It will feel a little cold on your teeth.

3．Breathe slowly through your nose.

4．Be still until it hardens.

5．I will remove the tray.

5 Quick Response
動画を見て、日本語に対する英語を瞬時に口頭で言いなさい。
瞬発力が大事です！

6 Handy Phrases
動画を見てとっさのひとことを確認しなさい。

濡れたエプロンを替えるときのひとこと。

Let me change your bib.（エプロンを替えましょう。）

7 Workout with Julia
動画を見て各器具の名称を写真の下に記入しなさい。
その後、英語の字幕を確認しながら実演動画を見なさい。

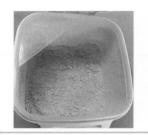
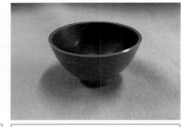
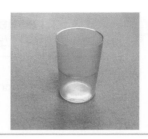

| 1 | 2 | 3 |

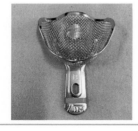
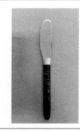

| 4 | 5 |

8 Dialogs
動画を見て各空欄に英単語 1 語を入れなさい。

Dialog 1：印象採得の手順

Hygienist: I will take an impression.

Patient: 　(　　　　　　　　　　) is it (　　　　　　　　　)?

Hygienist: It is necessary for making a model of your teeth.

Patient: 　I see.

Hygienist: Please relax, I will be back.

　　　　　 It will feel a little cold on your teeth.

Please open your mouth.

Breathe slowly through your nose.

Please be still until it hardens.

I will remove the tray.

Patient:　Phew!

Hygienist: Please rinse out your mouth.

Dialog 2：患者を安心させる

Hygienist: We are going to take an impression.

Patient:　Oh no!

Hygienist: Don't worry, I will do it as quickly as possible.

Patient:　But I (　　　　　　　　)(　　　　　　　　).

Hygienist: Don't worry, I have some good ideas.

　　　　　(plan A)

　　　　　Breathe slowly through your nose.

　　　　　(plan B)

　　　　　Hum a tune.

　　　　　(plan C)

　　　　　It is okay to drool.

9 Patient Interview Drill 13

▶巻末ドリルシート参照（p. 99-100）

a. 単語やフレーズの確認をしなさい。

available	入手可能な	**periodontal disease**	歯周病
bad breath	口臭	**either**	どちらも

b. 動画を見て患者さんの回答を問診表に書き込みなさい。

c. ペアを組んで歯科衛生士役と患者役に分かれて医療面接をしなさい。

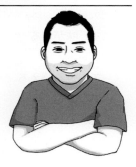

Lesson 14
Post-Treatment Instructions
処置後の注意

必要な動画を選んで
再生してください

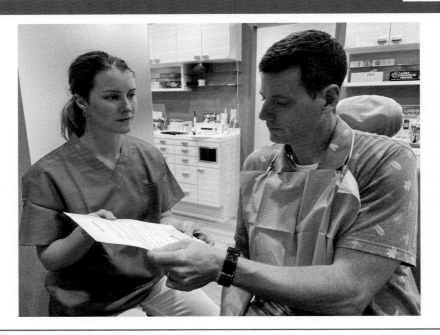

まあこのワンポイントアドバイス

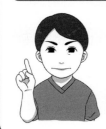

Minor surgical procedures are performed at dental clinics. Tooth extraction is one of these procedures. Many patients are worried about the pain during surgery, the bleeding from the surgical site, the type of medication, and the return to daily life such as eating or going to the gym. Appropriate information is extremely important both before and after the extraction. This will have a great effect on the prognosis.

1 Vocabulary
次の語を英語の場合は日本語に、日本語の場合は英語に直しなさい。

1．post-treatment	2．終わった	3．glad
4．味がする	5．ガーゼ	6．follow instructions
7．～を控える	8．wear off	9．surgical site
10．increase	11．blood flow	12．hot and spicy

2　Brian's Pronunciation Practice
動画の音声に続いて、リピートしなさい。

3　Brian's Pronunciation Tips
動画の音声に続いて、単語の発音練習をしなさい。

wo<u>rr</u>y　rr をしっかりと発音しましょう。

blood flow　形容詞＋名詞の場合は、続けて一気に発音しましょう。

al<u>co</u>hol　アルコールとは発音しません。co は「カ」に近い感じです。

4　Core Phrases
次の英文を和訳しなさい。

1．I will give you some post-treatment instructions.

2．The bleeding has been stopped.

3．Bite down on this gauze.

4．Please follow these instructions.

5．Refrain from eating and drinking.

6．Try not to touch the surgical site.

7．Refrain from activities that will increase blood flow.

5　Quick Response
動画を見て、日本語に対する英語を瞬時に口頭で言いなさい。
瞬発力が大事です！

6　Handy Phrases
動画を見てとっさのひとことを確認しなさい。

「施術後の注意」のひとこと。

　Don't bite your cheek.（頬を噛まないでくださいね。）

より丁寧に言いたかったら…

　Try not to … を動詞の前に付けてみましょう。

7　Workout with Julia
動画を見て薬の種類を英語で書きとりなさい。
次にそれぞれの薬の処方を聞き取って日本語で表に書きなさい。

	名称	用法	容量
1			
2			
3			
4			
5			

8　Dialogs
動画を見て各空欄に英単語1語を入れなさい。

Dialog 1：患者を安心させる（抜歯後）

Hygienist: We are finished.

Patient:　 I am glad that it is over.

Hygienist: I understand. I will give you some post-treatment instructions.

Patient:　 Before that, I (　　　　　　　) a (　　　　　　　).

Hygienist: Yes?

Patient:　 I still can (　　　　　　　) a little (　　　　　　　).

Hygienist: There is no need to worry.

　　　　　The bleeding has basically been stopped.

　　　　　If bleeding continues, bite down on this gauze for about 20 minutes.

Patient:　　I see.

Dialog 2：抜歯後の指導

Hygienist: Please follow these instructions.

　　　　　Refrain from eating and drinking until the anesthetic wears off.

　　　　　Try not to touch the surgical site with your tongue.

　　　　　Do not rinse out your mouth too much.

　　　　　It will cause bleeding.

　　　　　Please refrain from activities that will increase blood flow.

Patient:　　Can I (　　　　　　　　　) a (　　　　　　　　　)?

Hygienist: A shower would be better.

Patient:　　How about (　　　　　　　　)?

Hygienist: No. Do not drink alcohol.

　　　　　Do not eat hard food for several days.

　　　　　And please refrain from eating hot and spicy foods.

Patient:　　OK.

9 Patient Interview Drill 14
▶巻末ドリルシート参照（p.101-102）

a. 単語やフレーズの確認をしなさい。

discomfort　違和感　　　　　　　　　**worse**　よりひどい

weightlifting　ウエイトリフティング

b. 動画を見て患者さんの回答を問診表に書き込みなさい。

c. ペアを組んで歯科衛生士役と患者役に分かれて医療面接をしなさい。

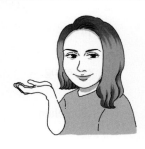

Lesson 15
Working with a Dental Technician
歯科技工士との協働

必要な動画を選んで
再生してください

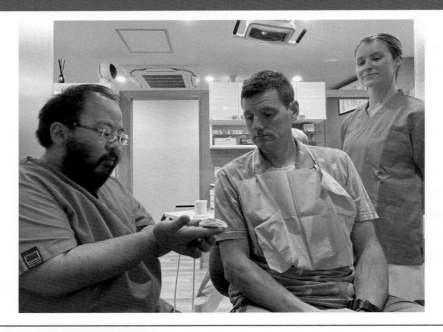

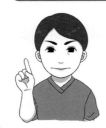

Team medicine plays an important role in providing treatment of high quality. Understanding the specialties of the other professionals participating in the team becomes necessary. At dental clinics, team medicine often involves cooperation among dentists, dental technicians, and dental hygienists. Sharing expertise to support patients will lead to treatment that is satisfying for all.

1 Vocabulary
次の語を英語の場合は日本語に、日本語の場合は英語に直しなさい。

1．dental technician	2．決める	3．shape
4．prefer	5．より白く	6．stand out
7．covering	8．front side	9．resin
10．porcelain	11．セラミックの	

2 Brian's Pronunciation Practice
動画の音声に続いて、リピートしなさい。

3 Brian's Pronunciation Tips
動画の音声に続いて、単語の発音練習をしなさい。

technician　一つ目の i を「イ」と発音せず、「イ」と「エ」の間の発音をしましょう。

resin　i を「イ」と発音せず、「イ」と「エ」の間の発音をしましょう。

ceramic　アクセントは a です。発音に注意しましょう。

4 Core Phrases
次の英文を和訳しなさい。

1．I am Mutti, your dental technician.

2．Let me check the color and shape.

3．A3 is the color of your teeth.

4．A2 will make it stand out.

5．There are several types of coverings.

6．The front side is resin and the back is metal.

5 Quick Response
動画を見て、日本語に対する英語を瞬時に口頭で言いなさい。
瞬発力が大事です！

6 Handy Phrases
動画を見てとっさのひとことを確認しなさい。

「施術後の注意」のひとこと。

    Don't touch it with your tongue.（舌で触らないようにしてください。）

より丁寧に言いたかったら…

    Try not to … を動詞の前に付けてみましょう。

7 Workout with Julia
動画を見て各名称を英語で書きとりなさい。

1		2	
3		4	
5		6	
7		8	
9		10	
11			

8 Dialogs
動画を見て各空欄に英単語1語を入れなさい。

Dialog 1：歯の色

Dental Hygienist: I will get the dental technician. We need to decide on the color.

Patient: Sure.

Dental Technician: Hi. I am Mutti, your technician.

Patient: Nice to meet you Mutti.

Dental Technician: Let me check the color and shape of your teeth. Please bite down.

    A3 is the color of your teeth.

Patient: I (   ) a (   ) color.

Dental Technician: A2 will make it stand out.

Dental Hygienist: I say he is right.

Patient: Yes, I guess so.

Dialog 2：歯のカバーの種類

Dental Hygienist:　There are several types of coverings for your front teeth.

Patient:　　　　　What are the differences?

Dental Hygienist:　I will call the dental technician. He will explain.

Patient:　　　　　Hey Mutti!

Dental Technician: Hello Brian.

Patient:　　　　　Is this (　　　　　　　　)(　　　　　　　　　) insurance?

Dental Technician: Yes, it is. The front side is resin and back is metal.

Patient:　　　　　This one looks more (　　　　　　　　) and (　　　　　　　　).

Dental Technician: Yes. The front side is porcelain.

Patient:　　　　　What about this?

Dental Technician: This one is totally ceramic.

Dental Hygienist:　However, it is not covered by insurance.

Patient:　　　　　Oh!

9　Patient Interview Drill 15　　　　▶巻末ドリルシート参照（p.103-104）

a.　動画を見て患者さんの回答を問診表に書き込みなさい。

b.　ドリルのフレーズ練習です。動画を見て発話しましょう。

　concerns　気になる（困った）こと　　　　**daily oral care**　日々の口腔ケア

c.　ペアを組んで歯科衛生士役と患者役に分かれて医療面接をしなさい。

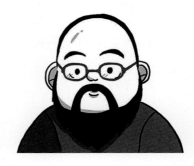

Lesson 16
Payment and Appointment
支払いと次回の予約

必要な動画を選んで
再生してください

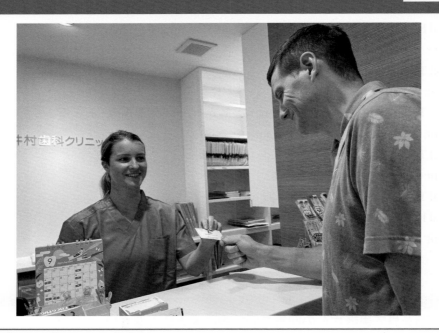

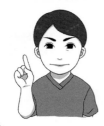

まあこのワンポイントアドバイス

After the treatment, the patient feels relieved to have the ordeal over. However, at the same time, they could be quite fatigued both physically and mentally. Some are in a rush to make it to their next appointment. Swiftly but surely explain the prescription, make sure the patient has their patient card returned, and reconfirm the date and time for the next visit. Finally, you can say to them, "Have a nice day!"

1 Vocabulary

次の語を英語の場合は日本語に、日本語の場合は英語に直しなさい。

1．payment

2．included

3．十万円

4．クレジットカード

5．bill

6．patient card

7．予約

8．available

9．prescription

10．pharmacy

2　Brian's Pronunciation Practice
動画の音声に続いて、リピートしなさい。

3　Brian's Pronunciation Tips
動画の音声に続いて、単語の発音練習をしなさい。

available　v の発音に注意しましょう。前歯で下唇を噛んで振動させる感じです。
prescription　tion は「ション」と発音しないように。
pharmacy　ph の箇所は f 音で発音しましょう。

4　Core Phrases
次の英文を和訳しなさい。

1．There is no payment for today.

2．It will be included in your next payment.

3．Here is your bill for today.

4．Your next treatment is 2 weeks from now.

5．These dates are available.

6．There is one just around the corner.

5　Quick Response
動画を見て、日本語に対する英語を瞬時に口頭で言いなさい。
瞬発力が大事です！

6 Handy Phrases
動画を見てとっさのひとことを確認しなさい。

ひざ掛けを外すときのひとこと。

Shall I remove the blanket?（ひざ掛けを取りましょうか。）

7 Workout with Julia

a. 動画を見て各名称を英語で書きとりなさい。

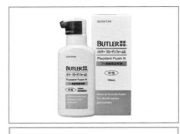

1

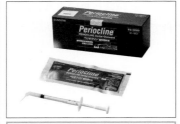

2

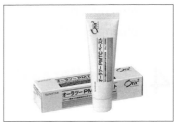

3

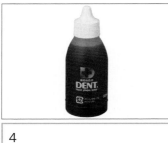

4

5

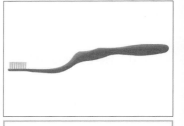

6

b. 動画を見て発音しなさい。

8 Dialogs
動画を見て各空欄に英単語1語を入れなさい。

Dialog 1：勘定は次の支払いで

Hygienist: There is no payment for today.

Patient:　　Really? Are you sure?

Hygienist: It will be included in your next payment.

Patient:　　I see. (　　　　　　　　)(　　　　　　　　) will I need?

Hygienist: We are going to fit your new ceramic crown.

　　　　　　As I explained before, it will be 100,000 yen before tax.

Patient:　　Yes, that's right...and I can use my credit card?

Hygienist: Of course.

Dialog 2：支払いとお見送り

Hygienist: Here is your bill for today.

And here is your patient card.

Patient:　　When is my next (　　　　　　　　)?

Hygienist: Your next treatment is 2 weeks from now.

These dates are available.

Patient:　　How about (　　　　　　　)(　　　　　　　) at

(　　　　　　　)(　　　　　　)?

Hygienist: Sure...and here is your prescription.

Patient:　　Where can I (　　　　　　) my prescription (　　　　　　)?

Hygienist: Any pharmacy.

Patient:　　I see.

Hygienist: There is one just around the corner.

Patient:　　Great.

9　Patient Interview Drill 16

▶巻末ドリルシート参照（p.105-106)

a.　動画を見て患者さんの回答を問診表に書き込みなさい。

b.　ドリルのフレーズ練習です。動画を見て発話しましょう。

sores　口内炎　　　　　　　　fatigued　疲れた

c.　ペアを組んで歯科衛生士役と患者役に分かれて医療面接をしなさい。

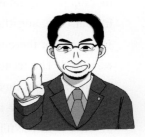

Dental Hygienists Around the World

4. The Netherlands

曽羽亜希子　奈良歯科衛生士専門学校元教務副主任

Wittenborg University of Applied Sciences English & Business Preparation Programme 在籍

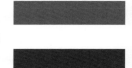

オランダ在住の曽羽亜希子さんに現地の歯科事情についてインタビューをしました。

Q1. How is the health insurance system in the Netherlands?

In the Netherlands, everyone is required to join a health insurance plan. Unlike Japan which has a national health insurance program, health care is provided by private companies. Dental care including orthodontic treatment for 18 year olds and under is covered by insurance.

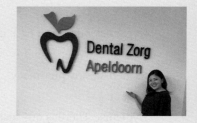

Q2. Which clinic did you visit?

I phoned a clinic called Dental Zorg Apeldooorn to make an appointment for my cracked dental filling. This bright and clean clinic offers a wide range of treatments such as periodontics, implants, esthetics, and orthodontics. All of the procedures are conducted in private treatment rooms. It should be noted that in the Netherlands, patients without appointments are not accepted unless it is a real emergency.

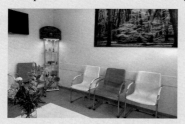
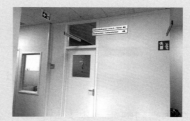

Q3. How was your treatment experience?

In the first visit, the dentist ("tandarts" in Dutch) interviewed, examined my condition, and took an x-ray. Showing the x-ray on the monitor, the dentist decided that the filling can be done without applying anesthetic. In the second visit, the utensils were already arranged as in the picture. An intern helped as an assistant. The dentist instructed me to signal if there is any pain. In that case, anesthetic will be applied. The procedures for resin filling were the same as in Japan except there was no rinsing out before and after the treatment. Instead, a dental suction was used. The treatment took about 15 minutes. Since all the preparations were completed before the visit, there was no waste of time in the treatment. As a result, it was a stress-free experience. The fee for the treatment was 40.73 euros for the interview and one x-ray picture in the first visit. The filling (including the adjacent tooth) cost 77.15 euros in the second visit.

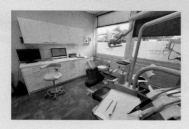 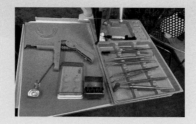

Q4. What kind of staff were there?

The staff included 2 dentists, 1 dental hygienist, 2 dental assistants, 1 receptionist, 1 manager, and 2 interns. Unfortunately, the hygienist who specializes in management for periodontal disease and cleanings was not present during my visit. According to the dentist, hygienists are qualified to apply local anesthetic to the patients. All through my treatment, there was a relaxed and friendly atmosphere. The dentist was even humming a tune while drilling. Since my appointment was fixed, there was plenty of time for explaining the procedures. They took time to answer all of my questions.

Text Message
Tue, 7 Jun, 08:36

U heeft binnenkort een afspraak met uw tandarts. Datum: wo 08/06, 13:05

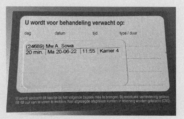

Q5. How are appointments made?

My first appointment was confirmed with a SMS message. The second appointment was printed out and pasted on to my patient card. In Japan, you sometimes have to wait even at an "appointment only" clinic. Often the staff gives the impression of being too busy to answer your questions. Furthermore, there still are many patients who visit without notice. In comparison, I discovered dental clinics in the Netherlands provide a stress-free environment for both patient and staff.

Vocabulary

utensils 器具   adjacent teeth 隣接歯

Patient Interview Drill 1

動画を見て、日本語で下の問診表を埋めなさい。　▶

↑動画再生はこちら

1．What seems to be the problem?　どうなさいましたか？
2．Where is the pain?　痛みはどこですか？
3．When did the pain start?　痛みはいつからですか？
4．What kind of pain is it?　どんな痛みですか？
5．Have you had a reaction to anesthetic?　麻酔に対してアレルギー反応を起こしたことはありますか？
6．Do you have any allergies?　アレルギーはありますか？
7．What are the side effects?　どのような副反応ですか？
8．Do you have any questions?　何かご質問はありますか？

問診表を埋められたら、裏面で答え合わせしましょう。

Patient Interview Drill 1

歯科衛生士役：動画のように英語で患者情報を聞いて書きとった後に英語で問診してみましょう。

患者役：自分の情報を英語で答えた後に問診表のとおり英語で回答してみましょう。

名前	
生年月日	
年齢	
血液型	

1．What seems to be the problem?　（歯科衛生士役）

　　I have a toothache.　（患者役）

2．Where is the pain?

　　It is in the bottom left.

3．When did the pain start?

　　It started one week ago.

4．What kind of pain is it?

　　It hurts when I drink something cold.

5．Have you had a reaction to anesthetic?

　　No, I haven't.

6．Do you have any allergies?

　　I am allergic to painkillers.

7．What are the side effects?

　　I get rashes all over.

8．Do you have any questions?

　　Is today's treatment covered by insurance?

Patient Interview Drill 2

動画を見て、日本語もしくは英語で下の問診表を埋めなさい。　▶

↑動画再生はこちら

1．How many times a day do you brush your teeth?　1日に何回歯を磨きますか？
2．When do you brush your teeth?　いつ歯を磨きますか？
3．How much time do you spend on each brushing?　毎回どれくらいの時間をかけますか？
4．Do you have any other oral care habits?　他にお口のお手入れはされていますか？
5．Do you smoke?　喫煙をされますか？
6．How often do you drink coffee, tea, or wine?　コーヒー、紅茶、ワインはどれくらい飲まれますか？
7．Do you eat between meals?　間食しますか？

問診表を埋められたら、裏面で答え合わせしましょう。

Patient Interview Drill 2

歯科衛生士役：動画のように英語で患者情報を聞いて書きとった後に英語で問診してみましょう。

患者役：自分の情報を英語で答えた後に問診表のとおり英語で回答してみましょう。

名前	
生年月日	
年齢	
血液型	

1．How many times a day do you brush your teeth? （歯科衛生士役）

　　I brush my teeth three times a day. （患者役）

2．When do you brush your teeth?

　　I brush my teeth after breakfast, after lunch, and before going to bed.

3．How much time do you spend on each brushing?

　　I spend about 3 minutes on each brushing.

4．Do you have any other oral care habits?

　　I use dental floss.

5．Do you smoke?

　　No, I don't.

6．How often do you drink coffee, tea, or wine?

　　I drink a lot of coffee.

7．Do you eat between meals?

　　No, I don't.

Patient Interview Drill 3

動画を見て、日本語もしくは英語で下の問診表を埋めなさい。　▶️　↑動画再生はこちら

1．What seems to be the problem?　どうなさいましたか？

2．Where is the pain?　痛みはどこですか？

3．When did the pain start?　痛みはいつからですか？

4．What kind of pain is it?　どんな痛みですか？

5．Did you take any painkillers?　痛み止めを服用しましたか？

6．Do you have any painkillers left?　痛み止めはまだありますか？

7．Have you ever had a reaction to anesthetic?　麻酔に対してアレルギー反応を起こしたことはありますか？

8．Do you have any questions?　何かご質問はありますか？

(Sure, we can.)

問診表を埋められたら、裏面で答え合わせしましょう。

Patient Interview Drill 3

歯科衛生士役：動画のように英語で患者情報を聞いて書きとった後に英語で問診してみましょう。

患者役：自分の情報を英語で答えた後に問診表のとおり英語で回答してみましょう。

名前	
生年月日	
年齢	
血液型	

1．What seems to be the problem？ （歯科衛生士役）

　　I have a toothache. It hurt so much that I couldn't sleep. （患者役）

2．Where is the pain?

　　It is in the upper right in the back.

3．When did the pain start?

　　It started a couple of days ago.

4．What kind of pain is it?

　　In the beginning it was a slight pain. Yesterday, it became a severe pain.

5．Did you take any painkillers?

　　Yes, I did.

6．Do you have any painkillers left?

　　No, I don't. I finished taking them all.

7．Have you ever had a reaction to anesthetic?

　　No, I haven't.

8．Do you have any questions?

　　Can you stop this pain now?

　　(Sure, we can.)

80

Patient Interview Drill 4

↑動画再生はこちら

動画を見て、日本語もしくは英語で下の問診表を埋めなさい。　▶

1．How many times a day do you brush your teeth?　1日に何回歯を磨きますか？

2．When do you brush your teeth?　いつ歯を磨きますか？

3．How much time do you spend on each brushing?　毎回どれくらいの時間をかけますか？

4．Do you have any other oral care habits?　他にお口のお手入れはされていますか？

5．Do you smoke?　喫煙をされますか？

6．How many cigarettes do you smoke a day?　1日に何本吸いますか？

7．How often do you drink coffee, tea, or wine?　コーヒー、紅茶、ワインはどれくらい飲まれますか？

8．Do you eat between meals?　間食しますか？

問診表を埋められたら、裏面で答え合わせしましょう。

キリトリ

キリトリ

Patient Interview Drill 4

歯科衛生士役：動画のように英語で患者情報を聞いて書きとった後に英語で問診してみましょう。

患者役：自分の情報を英語で答えた後に問診表のとおり英語で回答してみましょう。

名前	
生年月日	
年齢	
血液型	

1. How many times a day do you brush your teeth? （歯科衛生士役）

   I brush my teeth once a day. Sometimes, I don't brush at all. （患者役）

2. When do you brush your teeth?

   I brush in the morning.

3. How much time do you spend on each brushing?

   I am not sure. I don't pay much attention.

4. Do you have any other oral care habits?

   I always use a toothpick after meals.

5. Do you smoke?

   Yes, I do.

6. How many cigarettes do you smoke a day?

   I smoke about a pack a day.

7. How often do you drink coffee, tea, or wine?

   Not much. I drink a lot of beer.

8. Do you eat between meals?

   No, I don't.

Patient Interview Drill 5

動画を見て、日本語もしくは英語で下の問診表を埋めなさい。　▶

↑動画再生はこちら

1．What seems to be the problem?　どうなさいましたか？
2．Which tooth is it?　どの歯ですか？
3．When did this happen?　いつ起こりましたか？
4．What were you doing?　何をしていた時ですか？
5．Do you have any pain now?　今は痛みがありますか？
6．Do you have time for treatment today?　今日は治療のお時間ございますか？
7．Do you have health insurance?　健康保険に入っていますか？

問診表を埋められたら、裏面で答え合わせしましょう。

キリトリ

キリトリ

Patient Interview Drill 5

歯科衛生士役：動画のように英語で患者情報を聞いて書きとった後に英語で問診してみましょう。

患者役：自分の情報を英語で答えた後に問診表のとおり英語で回答してみましょう。

名前	
生年月日	
年齢	
血液型	

1．What seems to be the problem?　（歯科衛生士役）

　　I chipped my tooth.（患者役）

2．Which tooth is it?

　　The bottom left in the back.

3．When did this happen?

　　It happened this morning.

4．What were you doing?

　　I was eating granola.

5．Do you have any pain now?

　　No, I don't.

6．Do you have time for treatment today?

　　Yes, I have time.

7．Do you have health insurance?

　　Yes, I do.

Patient Interview Drill 6

↑動画再生はこちら

動画を見て、日本語もしくは英語で下の問診表を埋めなさい。

1．What kind of toothbrush do you use?　どのような歯ブラシをお使いですか？
2．Which do you use, soft, regular, or hard bristles?　柔らかい毛先、普通の毛先、固い毛先、どちらを使っていますか？
3．Why do you choose hard bristles?　なぜ固い毛先を選ぶのですか？
4．Where do you purchase your brushes?　歯ブラシはどちらで購入していますか？
5．Why do you buy online?　なぜオンラインで購入するのですか？
6．Have you ever received tooth-brushing instructions?　今まで歯磨き指導を受けたことはありますか？
7．Do you have time for instructions today?　今日は指導を受けるお時間はありますか？

問診表を埋められたら、裏面で答え合わせしましょう。

Patient Interview Drill 6

歯科衛生士役：動画のように英語で患者情報を聞いて書きとった後に英語で問診してみましょう。

患者役：自分の情報を英語で答えた後に問診表のとおり英語で回答してみましょう。

名前	
生年月日	
年齢	
血液型	

1．What kind of toothbrush do you use?（歯科衛生士役）

    I use a normal toothbrush.（患者役）

2．Which do you use, soft, regular, or hard bristles?

    I always choose hard bristles.

3．Why do you choose hard bristles?

    I think it cleans better.

4．Where do you purchase your brushes?

    I order online.

5．Why do you buy online?

    It is easier and cheaper that way.

6．Have you ever received tooth-brushing instructions?

    No, I haven't.

7．Do you have time for instructions today?

    I sure do.

キリトリ

Patient Interview Drill 7

↑動画再生はこちら

動画を見て、日本語もしくは英語で下の問診表を埋めなさい。　▶

1．What seems to be the problem?　どうなさいましたか？
2．Do you have it with you now?　今、お持ちですか？
3．Which tooth is it?　どの歯ですか？
4．When did it fall out?　いつ取れましたか？
5．What caused it to fall out?　何が原因で取れましたか？
6．Do you have any pain?　痛みはありますか？
7．Do you have time for treatment today?　今日は治療のお時間ございますか？
8．When did you get this crown?　このクラウンはいつ入れてもらったのですか？
9．Are you living in Japan now?　今は日本にお住まいですか？

問診表を埋められたら、裏面で答え合わせしましょう。

Patient Interview Drill 7

歯科衛生士役：動画のように英語で患者情報を聞いて書きとった後に英語で問診してみましょう。

患者役：自分の情報を英語で答えた後に問診表のとおり英語で回答してみましょう。

名前	
生年月日	
年齢	
血液型	

1．What seems to be the problem？　（歯科衛生士役）

　　My crown fell out.（患者役）

2．Do you have it with you now?

　　Here it is.

3．Which tooth is it?

　　It is the upper right...tooth in the back.

4．When did it fall out?

　　It fell out last night.

5．What caused it to fall out?

　　When I was eating something.

6．Do you have any pain?

　　Now, I don't.

7．Do you have time for treatment today?

　　Yes, I do.

8．When did you get this crown?

　　I got the crown in Boston...about 10 years ago.

9．Are you living in Japan now?

　　Yes, I am.

キリトリ　キリトリ

Patient Interview Drill 8

動画を見て、日本語もしくは英語で下の問診表を埋めなさい。　

↑動画再生はこちら

1．How many times a day do you brush?　1日に何回歯を磨きますか？

2．When do you brush your teeth?　いつ歯を磨きますか？

3．How much time do you spend on each brushing?　毎回どれくらいの時間をかけますか？

4．What kind of toothbrush do you use?　どのような歯ブラシをお使いですか？

5．How do you use them?　どのように使っていますか？

6．Do you have any questions concerning your brushing habits? 歯磨き習慣について何か聞きたいことはございますか？

7．It is ok to use both. I can give you more details later. Do you have time? 両方使っても問題ありません。後ほどもっと詳しく教えします。お時間ございますか？

問診表を埋められたら、裏面で答え合わせしましょう。

Patient Interview Drill 8

歯科衛生士役：動画のように英語で患者情報を聞いて書きとった後に英語で問診してみましょう。

患者役：自分の情報を英語で答えた後に問診表のとおり英語で回答してみましょう。

名前	
生年月日	
年齢	
血液型	

1．How many times a day do you brush?（歯科衛生士役）

   I brush three times a day.（患者役）

2．When do you brush your teeth?

   I brush in the morning, afternoon, and evening.

3．How much time do you spend on each brushing?

   It varies. Maybe 3 to 5 minutes.

4．What kind of toothbrush do you use?

   I use both manual and powered toothbrushes.

5．How do you use them?

   At home, I use the manual toothbrush. At my office, I use the powered one.

6．Do you have any questions concerning your brushing habits?

   Is what I am doing, ok?

7．It is ok to use both. I can give you more details later. Do you have time?

   Yes, I do.

キリトリ　キリトリ

Patient Interview Drill 9

↑動画再生はこちら

動画を見て、日本語もしくは英語で下の問診表を埋めなさい。　▶

1．Do you have any concerns in your daily oral care? 口腔ケアで気になる（困った）ことはありますか？
2．When do you brush your teeth?　いつ歯磨きしていますか？
3．Do you often drink coffee, tea, or wine?　コーヒー、紅茶、緑茶、ワインをよく飲まれますか？
4．What kind of toothbrush do you use?　どのような歯ブラシを使用されていますか？
5．What kind of toothpaste do you use?　どのような歯磨剤を使用されていますか？
6．Have you ever had stain removal at a dental clinic before? 　歯科医院でのステイン除去を受けたことがありますか？

問診表を埋められたら、裏面で答え合わせしましょう。

Patient Interview Drill 9

歯科衛生士役：動画のように英語で患者情報を聞いて書きとった後に英語で問診してみましょう。

患者役：自分の情報を英語で答えた後に問診表のとおり英語で回答してみましょう。

名前	
生年月日	
年齢	
血液型	

1．Do you have any concerns in your daily oral care?（歯科衛生士役）

No matter how much I brush, I get tooth stains.（患者役）

2．When do you brush your teeth?

Right after I wake up and before going to bed.

3．Do you often drink coffee, tea, or wine?

I drink 4 cups of coffee every day. In the weekends, I often drink wine.

4．What kind of toothbrush do you use?

I use a toothbrush with soft bristles.

5．What kind of toothpaste do you use?

I don't pay much attention.

6．Have you ever had stain removal at a dental clinic before?

Yes, about 6 months ago.

Patient Interview Drill 10

↑動画再生はこちら

動画を見て、日本語もしくは英語で下の問診表を埋めなさい。

1．What seems to be the problem?　どうなさいましたか？
2．Do you have it with you now?　今、お持ちですか？
3．Which tooth is it?　どの歯ですか？
4．When did it fall out?　いつ取れましたか？
5．What were you doing when it fell out?　取れた時は何をされていましたか？
6．Do you have any pain?　痛みはありますか？
7．Are you visiting Japan now?　日本を旅行中ですか？
8．When are you leaving?　お帰りはいつですか？ 　　(Oh my!　あら！)

問診表を埋められたら、裏面で答え合わせしましょう。

Patient Interview Drill 10

歯科衛生士役：動画のように英語で患者情報を聞いて書きとった後に英語で問診してみましょう。

患者役：自分の情報を英語で答えた後に問診表のとおり英語で回答してみましょう。

名前	
生年月日	
年齢	
血液型	

1．What seems to be the problem?　（歯科衛生士役）

　　My filling came off.（患者役）

2．Do you have it with you now?

　　I might have swallowed it.

3．Which tooth is it?

　　It is in the upper left in the back.

4．When did it fall out?

　　It fell out just a while ago.

5．What were you doing when it fell out?

　　I was eating mochi.

6．Do you have any pain?

　　Yes, when I drink something cold.

7．Are you visiting Japan now?

　　Yes, I am.

8．When are you leaving?

　　Tomorrow.

　　(Oh my!)

Patient Interview Drill 11

動画を見て、日本語もしくは英語で下の問診表を埋めなさい。　▶️　↑動画再生はこちら

1．Are you using any oral care products?　補助的清掃用具は使用していますか？

2．When did you start using it?　いつから使用していますか？

3．What made you start?　始めたきっかけは何ですか？

4．What type are you using?　どんなタイプの物を使用していますか？

5．When do you use it?　いつ使用していますか？

6．Have you experienced any problems?　使用していて困っていることはありますか？

7．I don't think so. I will show you how to use it.　よくないと思います。使い方を教えます。

問診表を埋められたら、裏面で答え合わせしましょう。

Patient Interview Drill 11

歯科衛生士役：動画のように英語で患者情報を聞いて書きとった後に英語で問診してみましょう。

患者役：自分の情報を英語で答えた後に問診表のとおり英語で回答してみましょう。

名前	
生年月日	
年齢	
血液型	

1．Are you using any oral care products?（歯科衛生士役）

    Yes, I use dental floss.（患者役）

2．When did you start using it?

    I started using it 6 months ago.

3．What made you start?

    My dentist recommended it.

4．What type are you using?

    It is straight with a grip.

5．When do you use it?

    Only when something is stuck between my teeth.

6．Have you experienced any problems?

    Sometimes there is bleeding. Is that ok?

7．I don't think so. I will show you how to use it.

    Yes, please.

キリトリ

キリトリ

Patient Interview Drill 12

動画を見て、日本語もしくは英語で下の問診表を埋めなさい。　▶

↑動画再生はこちら

1．What seems to be the problem?　どうなさいましたか？

2．Where is the swelling?　どこが腫れていますか？

3．When did the swelling start?　いつから腫れだしましたか？

4．Do you have any pain?　痛みはありますか？

5．When does it hurt?　いつ痛みますか？

6．Are you allergic to painkillers or antibiotics?　痛み止めや抗生剤にアレルギーはありますか？

7．Do you have health insurance?　健康保険に入っていますか？

問診表を埋められたら、裏面で答え合わせしましょう。

Patient Interview Drill 12

歯科衛生士役：動画のように英語で患者情報を聞いて書きとった後に英語で問診してみましょう。

患者役：自分の情報を英語で答えた後に問診表のとおり英語で回答してみましょう。

名前	
生年月日	
年齢	
血液型	

1．What seems to be the problem?　（歯科衛生士役）

　　My gums are swollen.（患者役）

2．Where is the swelling?

　　It is in my bottom right.

3．When did the swelling start?

　　It started about a week ago.

4．Do you have any pain?

　　Yes, I do.

5．When does it hurt?

　　When I eat and when I brush my teeth.

6．Are you allergic to painkillers or antibiotics?

　　No, I am not.

7．Do you have health insurance?

　　Oops! I forgot to bring it today.

Patient Interview Drill 13

動画を見て、日本語もしくは英語で下の問診表を埋めなさい。　▶️　↑動画再生はこちら

1．Do you have any concerns in your daily oral care?　口腔ケアで気になる（困った）ことはありますか？
2．What kind are you using now?　今はどのような歯磨剤を使用されていますか？
3．Have you experienced any problems with it?　使用していて問題があるのですか？
4．Is there anything that bothers you now?　今、お口の中に気になることはありますか？
5．Any other concerns?　他にありますか？
6．Do you often drink coffee, tea, or wine?　コーヒー、紅茶、緑茶、ワインをよく飲まれますか？

問診表を埋められたら、裏面で答え合わせしましょう。

Patient Interview Drill 13

歯科衛生士役：動画のように英語で患者情報を聞いて書きとった後に英語で問診してみましょう。

患者役：自分の情報を英語で答えた後に問診表のとおり英語で回答してみましょう。

名前	
生年月日	
年齢	
血液型	

1．Do you have any concerns in your daily oral care?（歯科衛生士役）

I wish to know what kind of toothpaste I should use.（患者役）

2．What kind are you using now?

I am using a toothpaste recommended by my dentist.

3．Have you experienced any problems with it?

No, just that it is not available in Japan.

4．Is there anything that bothers you now?

I am worried about periodontal disease.

5．Any other concerns?

I am also worried about my bad breath.

6．Do you often drink coffee, tea, or wine?

I don't drink much of either.

キリトリ

Patient Interview Drill 14

動画を見て、日本語もしくは英語で下の問診表を埋めなさい。　▶

↑動画再生はこちら

１．What seems to be the problem?　どうなさいましたか？
２．Do you have any pain?　痛みはありますか？
３．When did the discomfort start?　いつから違和感がありましたか？
４．Have you had jaw problems before?　今まで顎のトラブルはございましたか？
５．Do you clench your teeth often?　よく歯を食いしばりますか？
６．Does anyone say you grind your teeth when you sleep? 　寝ている時に歯ぎしりをすると言われたことはありますか？
７．Do you have health insurance?　健康保険に入っていますか？

問診表を埋められたら、裏面で答え合わせしましょう。

キリトリ

キリトリ

Patient Interview Drill 14

歯科衛生士役：動画のように英語で患者情報を聞いて書きとった後に英語で問診してみましょう。

患者役：自分の情報を英語で答えた後に問診表のとおり英語で回答してみましょう。

名前	
生年月日	
年齢	
血液型	

1．What seems to be the problem?　（歯科衛生士役）

　　I have discomfort in my jaws.（患者役）

2．Do you have any pain?

　　No, I don't.

3．When did the discomfort start?

　　It started about 1 year ago. However, it started to get worse last week.

4．Have you had jaw problems before?

　　No, I haven't.

5．Do you clench your teeth often?

　　I always do weight lifting at the gym. Maybe then.

6．Does anyone say you grind your teeth when you sleep?

　　Yes, my wife says so.

7．Do you have health insurance?

　　Yes, I do.

Patient Interview Drill 15

動画を見て、日本語もしくは英語で下の問診表を埋めなさい。　▶

↑動画再生はこちら

1．Do you have any concerns in your daily oral care?　口腔ケアで気になる（困った）ことはありますか？
2．Where is the pain?　どこが痛みますか？
3．What kind of pain is it?　どのような痛みですか？
4．Is there any pain when you are not brushing?　歯磨き以外の時にも痛みはありますか？
5．　What kind of toothbrush are you using?　どのような歯ブラシを使用していますか？
6．What kind of toothpaste are you using?　どのような歯磨剤を使用していますか？

問診表を埋められたら、裏面で答え合わせしましょう。

Patient Interview Drill 15

歯科衛生士役：動画のように英語で患者情報を聞いて書きとった後に英語で問診してみましょう。

患者役：自分の情報を英語で答えた後に問診表のとおり英語で回答してみましょう。

名前	
生年月日	
年齢	
血液型	

1．Do you have any concerns in your daily oral care?（歯科衛生士役）

   I experience pain during tooth brushing.（患者役）

2．Where is the pain?

   Several places but especially in my upper right.

3．What kind of pain is it?

   There is a sharp pain when I brush.

4．Is there any pain when you are not brushing?

   It hurts when I drink something cold.

5．What kind of toothbrush are you using?

   I use a toothbrush with hard bristles because it cleans better.

6．What kind of toothpaste are you using?

   I use whitening toothpaste because I am concerned about my tooth stains.

Patient Interview Drill 16

動画を見て、日本語もしくは英語で下の問診表を埋めなさい。　▶️

↑動画再生はこちら

1．What seems to be the problem?　どうなさいましたか？
2．Where is it?　どこですか？
3．When did it start?　いつからですか？
4．How is the pain?　痛みはどうですか？
5．Do you often get sores?　よく口内炎になりますか？
6．Do you feel fatigued recently?　最近、疲れを感じていますか？
7．Were you able to eat?　食事はできました？
8．Do you have health insurance?　健康保険に入っていますか？

問診表を埋められたら、裏面で答え合わせしましょう。

Patient Interview Drill 16

歯科衛生士役：動画のように英語で患者情報を聞いて書きとった後に英語で問診してみましょう。
患者役：自分の情報を英語で答えた後に問診表のとおり英語で回答してみましょう。

名前	
生年月日	
年齢	
血液型	

1．What seems to be the problem?　（歯科衛生士役）

　　I have a large canker sore. I have trouble eating.（患者役）

2．Where is it?

　　It is behind my lower lip.

3．When did it start?

　　It started about 3 days ago.

4．How is the pain?

　　It especially hurts when I eat.

5．Do you often get sores?

　　Yes, I do.

6．Do you feel fatigued recently?

　　Yes, very much. Actually, I had a fever all last week.

7．Were you able to eat?

　　Not much.

8．Do you have health insurance?

　　Yes, I do.

キリトリ

キリトリ

この度は弊社の書籍をご購入いただき、誠にありがとうございました。
本書籍に掲載内容の更新や訂正があった際は、弊社ホームページ「追加情報」
にてお知らせいたします。下記のURLまたはQRコードをご利用ください。

https://www.nagasueshoten.co.jp/extra.html

歯科衛生士英語ワークブック　　　　　　　　　　　　　　ISBN 978-4-8160-1414-7

© 2023. 1. 20　第1版　第1刷

監　　修	山本一世	
編　　著	藤田淳一	
発 行 者	永末英樹	
印　　刷	創栄図書印刷 株式会社	
製　　本	新生製本 株式会社	

発行所　株式会社　永末書店

〒602-8446　京都市上京区五辻通大宮西入五辻町 69-2
（本社）電話 075-415-7280　FAX 075-415-7290
永末書店 ホームページ　https://www.nagasueshoten.co.jp